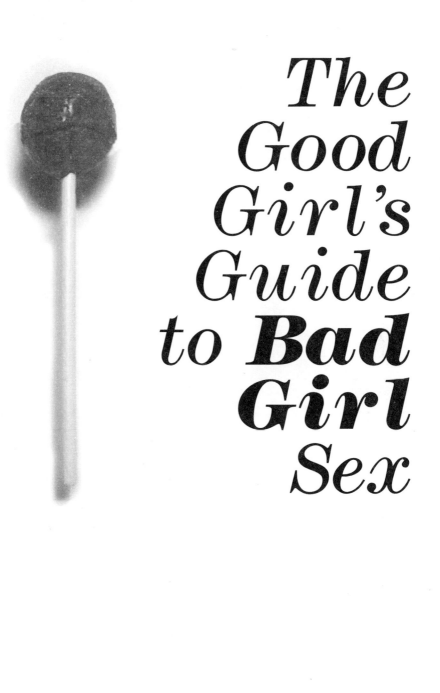

The Good Girl's Guide to **Bad Girl** Sex

*The Good Girl's Guide to **Bad Girl Sex***

An Indispensable Resource for Pleasure and Seduction

Barbara Keesling, Ph.D.

M. Evans and Company, Inc.
New York

M. Evans and Company, Inc.
216 East 49th Street
New York, New York 10017

Library of Congress Cataloging-in-Publication Data

Keesling, Barbara.
  The good girl's guide to bad girl sex / by Barbara Keesling.
    p.   cm.
  Includes index.
  ISBN 0-87131-934-9
  1. Women—Sexual behavior. 2. Women—Psychology. 3. Sex (Psychology).
I. Title.
HQ29 .K444 2001
306.7'082—dc21   2001023174

Book design and typesetting by Rik Lain Schell

Printed in the United States of America

9   8   7   6   5

To all the Good Girls who are ready for some BAD

Contents

Introduction

Every good girl I have ever known wishes somewhere in her heart that she could be just a little bit bad. She wishes she could turn a few heads with the way she walks, raise a few eyebrows with the way she talks, raise a man's temperature when she enters the room, and leave him breathless when she exits.

But that isn't how most of us were raised. If you are like most of the women I know, and I'm guessing that you are, you were probably raised to do the right things and to say the right things. To be respectful. And kind. And decent. And modest. To be, first and foremost, always a "lady." In short, to be a Good Girl.

The place you needed to be the epitome of "good"—the most careful and ladylike of all—was the place where it was most dangerous to be the least bit "bad": behind closed doors in the arms of a man. Why? Because making love should be something lovely and special and soft and gentle and quiet and private and very, very *feminine*—something to be shared in a discreet and loving way in the quiet evening hours with the one you love. This was the picture society painted for most of us, and to bring that idealized picture to life, you had to be *good*.

Did Good Girls have sex? Of course they did. Good Girls could even enjoy sex, as long as they didn't enjoy it *too* much. But Good Girls didn't crave sex. And Good Girls didn't breathe sex. Good Girls certainly didn't exude sex and Good Girls didn't *live* sex. All of that was for the Bad Girls.

Oh, those Bad Girls. You know them well. For years you have listened to their stories and watched them turn heads. How did they get to be so sexy? How did they get to be so hot? How did they get to be so free? How did they get to be so *bad*? And what does that feel like? If you're like me, you have asked yourself these questions. My goal is to help you find the answers—answers you can live with and love with.

My name is Barbara Keesling, and I am a sex therapist in private practice in Southern California. I have been a sex therapist for over ten years. Before receiving my doctorate I worked for many years as a professional surrogate partner—someone who assists a sex therapist in a clinical setting to help the therapist's patients work through sexual obstacles. Clearly, I have spent a great deal of time in the pursuit of sexual understanding, but don't let that fool you into thinking that I was "born to be bad." Like most women, I have struggled to find my sexual power. For many years I was just like you: a really Good Girl who wanted to be bad. I had to learn everything that you will need to learn, and I think that makes me a uniquely qualified guide. Today I am a very different woman than I was back then—I am, as they say, "as bad as I wanna be." I hope that my personal story, along with the many other stories I will be sharing in this book, will give you support and some genuine inspiration.

If you have been a Good Girl all of your life, it may not be all that easy to suddenly be "bad." You have it in you—every woman has that special something in her—that, I'm sure of. It may take a little time to find it and it may take a little practice to learn how to use it, but you're going to find it. You are going to feel it. You are going to learn how to use it really soon. It doesn't take long once you start looking for it and you can start looking right now by just turning the page.

If you have picked up this book you are ready for a change, and you need that change right now! You need to be sexy. You need to be wicked. You need to be lustful. You need to be wild; so wild you could scream. Bottom line: *You need to be bad.* You need to be bad so that sex can feel good. So it can feel fabulous. Mind-blowing. Hot as Hades. You owe this to yourself—and it's time you got what you deserve.

The Good Girl's Guide to Bad Girl Sex is written just for you. It doesn't matter if you're twenty-five or fifty-five. It doesn't matter if

Introduction

you're married or single. It doesn't matter if you're in love or in lust. All that matters is that you want it *bad*. I know what your fears are and I know your concerns, but I also know that you need to be bad. Life is too short to waste it being good. It's time for you to learn to enjoy what all the Bad Girls know.

Chapter 1

Bad Girls Feel Good about Being Bad

Fact: *Sex is not a four-letter word.*

When Jane was a teenager, she would often go without a bra. She was proud of her small, perfectly shaped bosom. She also enjoyed the way fabrics felt against her skin; the smooth, cool glide of cotton across her chest or the luxurious caress of her favorite satin blouse.

This small but important practice was just enough to keep Jane in touch with her body and her growing awareness of herself as a sexual being. Although she was still a virgin, she was beginning to understand the power that a sexually enlivened woman possesses—as was demonstrated by the appreciative glances she would sometimes garner from her male classmates.

All that came to a screeching halt the day Jane's mother took her shopping for some new clothes and discovered in the dressing room that her daughter was not wearing a bra. "Are you out of your mind? What kind of message do you think that sends to people? Do you want boys to think that you're loose? That you're cheap? That you're a tramp? Now you march out there and come back with an armful of brassieres! Braless indeed!" Thus began Jane's all too lengthy slide into "Good-Girlhood." Her mother's unfortunate harangue haunted Jane for years to come. It influenced her behavior regarding the clothes she bought, the movies she saw, the language she used, even the way she looked at herself in the mirror. Jane's mother's comment was so loaded with threat and innuendo that Jane's Bad Girl took a ten-year sabbatical!

Although the set up and the particulars may be very different, I bet you could tell a story that sounds a whole lot like Jane's. Do you remember the first time your budding sexuality was trampled on, dismissed, or similarly snuffed out? So many women go through life apologizing for their sexual impulses and talking themselves out of their own desires. The feelings are there. The need is there. The drive is there. But it all creates such discomfort. Why? Because, "A Good Girl isn't supposed to be that *sexual*." That's what we've been told, and, like good little girls, we comply.

Are You Your Own Worst Sexual Enemy?

When we are young we are chaste, and the adults we come in contact with treat us accordingly—our parents, siblings, peers, teachers, neighbors, clergy, etc. The problem is, as we get older we have no one "in charge" to help us make the transition into sexual beings. It's funny how easy it seems to be to talk to young girls about what they shouldn't do in terms of dressing provocatively, wearing makeup, and so on. It's much harder to talk about how to do things in an attractive, sophisticated, and sexy manner—in short, how to develop into a sexually healthy woman. Usually we have to learn this on our own.

Sexuality Is Always Welcome in the Bad Girl's World

Bad Girls have no shame. I want you to memorize that sentence right now because it is going to be one of your new personal mantras. Bad Girls have no shame. What does that mean? It means that they are proud of who they are and what they feel. They *love* being bad (in fact they live for it!) and they have no interest in hiding that. Bad Girls are not ashamed to feel desire. They are not ashamed to admit their desire or to act on it. Now doesn't that make you want to shout "Sign me up!"?

Bad Girls announce their intentions. They announce them with the way they walk, the way they talk, and the way they dress and undress. They announce their intentions when they stand up, when they sit down, when they eat, and when they smile. What are a Bad Girl's intentions? *To be hot, to be in touch, and to be fully sexually alive with herself and with her sexual partner.* Clear, powerful, to the point, and very, very Bad. Yet they express this in a way that is never cheap, never trashy, never tawdry. Bad Girls feel sexy and fabulous and desirable. They don't *need* to be "good"; they love how it feels being bad.

Let's look at those intentions again: "To be hot, to be in touch, and to be fully sexually alive with her sexual partner." What are you thinking to yourself right now? Are you thinking, "I want to be hot, I want to be in touch, I want to be fully sexually alive. I have the same intentions!" I think you are, and I hope you are, yet there is a world of difference between having those intentions and living those intentions out loud. Bad Girls live out loud. That's what sets them apart. Don't let that discourage you. I have every reason to believe that you are ready to turn up your own personal volume. Maybe just a little at first, and then a little more every time as you get increasingly comfortable. I believe you are ready. And it doesn't take much to get you started. Before we do any more shouting, however, I want to make a few other things clear.

Bad Girls come in all shapes, sizes, heights, weights, and colors. It's what's inside that counts the most. A bad-to-the-bone Bad Girl isn't rocked by this week's hemline or bullied by last week's "must-have" color. Bad goes deeper than that, Bad is more confident than that, Bad is more anchored than that, and I'm going to help you find that anchor.

Bad can't be bought and it can't be faked for long. Bad *can* be uncovered, dusted off, shined up, honed, and enhanced. Bad has a sense of humor. Bad isn't rigid; Bad is flexible and can go with the flow when necessary. The great thing about Bad is, once it's yours and you really own it, *no one* can take it away from you. It becomes as much a part of you as your unerring sense of direction, your love of black and white movies, or your ability to curl your tongue.

7

But Bad is a muscle, and like any muscle, you have to use it if you want to keep it vibrant and strong. Bad *will* go to sleep on you if it gets stashed away up in the proverbial old attic, left to languish in a dusty old trunk that never sees the light of day.

Does that make you wonder if you ever really had it to stash away in the first place? Oh, you had it all right. At some point in your life, in one form or another, *you were Bad*. How do I know? Because if you never had it, you wouldn't be missing it now—and you must be missing it, or you wouldn't be trying to get it back! Okay, so it may have been brief—the merest whiff or glimpse of the Bad Girl within, but you saw her and you liked what you saw; you liked how you felt and you liked who you were.

It's Time to Reclaim the Bad Girl Within

Sexual power can be very threatening to those around you who'd prefer it if you stayed in your Good Girl role. If your Bad Girl wasn't met with open arms when she first made her debut (and my *very* educated guess is that she wasn't!), she could easily have been shamed, shouted, and shaken back into seclusion. Perhaps you saw her from time to time in weird dreams, in an occasional guilty fantasy, or in some experimental behavior you once indulged in (and have been trying very hard to forget). This is all very typical when the Bad Girl goes into hiding.

So how do we get that Bad Girl out of hiding? Frankly, I think you've already started. How? Just by reading these first few pages and not pushing the ideas away. So congratulations—you've already taken a step. As this chapter continues, we're going to take a few more vital first steps to get you on the path to *healthy desire*—that place where shame is never welcome. Getting to the source of your resistance is our goal here. We're going to look at damaging, fearful old messages and behaviors and replace them with something new, something sexy, something smoldering. . . . You can't be bad if you don't *love* being bad, and the place to start is deep inside where your greatest resistance still stands.

It's time to rewrite some of those self-defeating sexual programs and shed that Good Girl skin. Sexual desire is nothing to be ashamed of, even if (*especially* if) it is completely unbridled. Sexual desire should be celebrated, and the party is about to start.

Stop the Madness!

Fact: *A healthy sexual appetite is a natural and beautiful thing.*

Looking back on my sexual development, I thank my lucky stars that I came of age during a very narrow window of time, now affectionately referred to as "the '70s." It was after the women's libbers had made their mark and the 1960s had loosened everything up, but it was before the problematic 1980s when men and women had to worry about AIDS, and men started to care more about Wall Street and putting another stock in their portfolio than putting a notch in the bedpost (thanks for nothing, Michael Douglas!).

During the serendipitous '70s, it was absolutely okay for a woman to sleep with whomever she wanted, whenever she wanted. Believe me when I tell you that I was no Spice Girl at the time, either. No way— not with the big glasses, the extra fifteen pounds, and the slight over- bite I was sporting back then. I can't say I was being bad, even though I was having sex, because it was almost by default, instead of by design.

At age 24, I trained to be a surrogate partner. A sexual surrogate works with a sex therapist and his/her patient in a controlled, therapeu- tic environment. Together, the therapist and the surrogate help the patient with sexual problems he or she may be struggling with. It was at this time in my life that the doors to Badness first cracked open for me, giving me a glimpse into a world I could scarcely have dreamed existed. In addition to learning specific sexual techniques for my job that had the unexpected side effect of helping *me* access more of my sexuality, I had the rare opportunity to interview and interact with older, more experienced professional surrogates who were in full Bad Girl bloom. At work, these women were skilled professionals who adhered to a very strict code of appropriate conduct, but after hours it was a very differ- ent story. Many of these women showed themselves to have sexual appetites that were as natural, as dependable, and as guiltlessly satisfied as the need for a good meal. In order to stimulate the physical appetite, you whet it with a delicious, aromatic appetizer. If you don't eat regu- larly, your stomach shrinks and your capacity for food diminishes. Bland, tasteless food may fill you up, but it certainly won't satisfy you or

9

excite your taste buds. In fact, a healthy sexual appetite is remarkably similar to a healthy physical appetite:

- In order to stimulate the sexual appetite, you whet it with fantasy, visualization and foreplay.
- If you are not stoking your sexual fires on a regular basis, the fire can die out, and then your capacity for enjoying sex will diminish.
- There's sex and then there's SEX. A fully evolved Bad Girl can have an epic sexual encounter in ten minutes, whereas a woman stuck in her Good Girl can have intercourse for an hour and still be left feeling unfulfilled.

Do you apologize for having a physical appetite? For needing to eat? Of course you don't. Your physical appetite is a naturally occurring and integral part of who you are as a human being. Not only is it vital to your survival, but hopefully, it is also a source of pleasure and enjoyment for you.

Now ask yourself this: Do you apologize for having a *sexual* appetite? Do you deny *having* a sexual appetite? Why? Do you know many men who apologize for their sexual appetites? In fact, a man who states he needs sex often—once or more a day, for example—is considered a *stud,* and other men look at him with a certain amount of awe and respect. A woman making a similar claim to a group of her peers is often labeled sick, a slut, or a freak; even if she happens to be married! Why in the world should women be any less "hungry" than men? If you think about it in purely biological terms, it doesn't make any sense that we would be less hungry; any more so than we should experience any fewer hunger pangs when faced with a shortage of food.

It is important that you start viewing your sexual appetite similarly to your physical appetite. Your sexual hunger is as *natural* as your physical hunger. Your sexual hunger is an innate part of who you are as a human being. Can you die from not having great Bad Girl sex? Not exactly, but every time you have sex and you know it isn't as hot, as horny, as "bad" as you know it could be, I believe a little piece of you fades away. Your sexual hunger, vitality, and fulfillment are crucial contributors to your existing as a fully alive, fully functioning, and fully realized woman. It's as obvious as the clitoris between your legs that sex should be a source of great pleasure and enjoyment for you.

Bad Girls Feel Good about Being Bad

So, I ask you again: What's stopping you? What's getting in your way? Why aren't you *Bad?* My guess is that it's "the Bad Girl blockade."

Myths and Misconceptions: The Bad Girl Blockade

What is the first mental image that pops into your head when you think of the phrase "Bad Girl"? Be honest here, because it's going to help you break through to the other side of your sexuality.

- Is it a trashy streetwalker?
- Someone with a drug or alcohol problem who doesn't remember from one night to the next who she's been with?
- Or maybe something milder—just a woman with no self control. Someone who can't say "no" to anyone?
- Is a Bad Girl someone with low self-esteem who looks for validation through having lots of indiscriminate sex?
- Or maybe it's someone who can't get off unless she's sleeping with some other woman's man?

If these are the kinds of images that first come to mind when you conjure up a Bad Girl, it's no wonder you've avoided your own Bad Girl self. This little list I've made for you contains just *some* of the brash statements I've heard from my students and patients when I've asked them to define a Bad Girl for me. But guess what? They're way off base. These are *not* the definitions of a Bad Girl. These are descriptions of *troubled* girls. They are descriptions of women who act out varying degrees of emotional problems through sex—women who need professional help (and not just from a sex therapist). That's sad, not bad; yet these statements reflect classic Bad Girl stereotypes that many women hold dear.

The biggest challenge I face as the author of this book, and the biggest hurdle you have to overcome as a "Bad-Girl-in-training" is the challenge of erasing these Bad Girl stereotypes and reprogramming your brain with some new, healthy, basic information. Information like this: **Being bad means having it good.** And like this: **Being a "Good**

Girl" is being a *bored* girl (and let's face it, when we're bored, we're usually boring, too!).

Are you with me so far? Great. Now here is a short, but very important list of just some of the things a *true* Bad Girl is *not*.

Being Bad Does NOT Mean

- Being immoral or illegal
- Acting cheap
- Being pornographic or obscene in public
- Behaving dangerously or acting recklessly
- Being a sexual contortionist
- Demeaning yourself or degrading yourself with your sexual behavior
- Being indiscriminate with your sexual partners

What other negative behaviors or character traits do you associate with being a Bad Girl? It's important to flush some of these ideas out of the brush. Think back: was there a neighborhood "Bad Girl" when you were growing up? What was she like? Was she *troubled*, or was she just *bad*? How did you know she was bad? Was it just a rumor, or was it something you could *feel*? What was her name? I bet you can still remember it, can't you? She both fascinated and repelled you, intrigued and disturbed you, didn't she? She was mysterious and obvious all at the same time. Maybe she was a true, powerful, and healthy Bad Girl and maybe she wasn't. You just knew that she was breaking taboos; you knew she had access to a part of herself that *you* were not getting much encouragement to explore from anyone in *your* personal circle.

Well, call me Glinda the Good Witch, because with your consent and cooperation, we're going to rediscover everything *good* about being truly *bad*. Using this book as my magic wand, I promise to give you the permission, provide you with the encouragement, and lead you down the yellow brick road to meet your personal "Wizardress of Aahs," your neglected "Goddess of Gasps," and your inner "Baroness of Badness."

So click those ruby red Manolo Blahnik stilettos together three times and repeat after me: *"There's nothing wrong with being bad, there's nothing wrong with being bad, there's nothing wrong with being bad."*

Bad Girls Feel Good about Being Bad

I'm trying to put a smile on your face here, but I'm also completely serious. A grown woman stuck in her "Good Girl" is not a laughing matter. Having zero access to your inner "bad" diminishes your quality of life. It crushes your spirit. It can also take a heavy toll on your relationships; both in and out of bed.

The changes I have seen take place in a woman's life when she sheds her out-dated, prohibitive sexual patterns and embraces a "new world order" where she is free to express her sexuality to its fullest, reach far beyond the bedroom. These changes infuse every aspect of her life. She becomes more powerful in her work, more effective in her communication, and more confident in her abilities. I want those kinds of positive changes for you, too. Being bad is good for you; and I'm going to prove it.

What's So Good about Being Bad?

Okay. We've taken a look at some of the things that being Bad *isn't*. Now let's start exploring just exactly what being Bad *is*. Among other things,

Being Bad Means

- Loving sex!
- Being sexually confident
- Being physically uninhibited
- Feeling sexual hunger and knowing how to feed it
- Being assertive and unashamed
- Being fully integrated
- Being intensely orgasmic

Now that's not so awful, is it? In fact, I'll bet it sounds pretty good! I wish I could cut this list out of the page right now and paste it on your favorite mirror because you deserve to be reminded of this sexual reality every day. It doesn't sound "made up," or false, unnatural, or undoable, does it? At worst, it just sounds kind of foreign; like a country you've heard of, but never visited before. The good news is, you're holding your passport in your hands and I've just stamped it. The only bad news is that the journey doesn't happen overnight. But I promise you this: The scenery along the way is spectacular and you'll have memories that will last a lifetime. So take a deep breath and get comfortable. Next stop, Wonderland. . . .

Through the Looking Glass

Have you ever stopped to wonder how your sexuality was formed? Where it came from? Why it is the way it is? These are very important questions. Yet a lot of women—the majority of women—never give questions like this a passing thought. They just have sex. But these are very important questions—questions that are going to spark some memories, get you thinking seriously about your sexual power, and probably open your eyes to some aspects of your sexual self to which you've never given a passing thought.

Important as these questions are, however, they're not half as important as your answers. Not *my* answers. Yours. It is my fervent hope and wish that your answers will, at the very *least,* surprise you. Some will amuse you. Some will confuse you. Some, quite possibly, may even appall you. But what I'm really hoping is that some will anger you— anger you to the point where you are motivated to break those old Good Girl chains. Motivated to become the lean, mean, Bad Girl machine you know you want to be. Motivated to *rediscover* and *reclaim* your natural sexual birthright. Motivated to step into your power and get fully comfortable in your Baddest sexual self.

Go Ask Alice . . .

Like Alice in Wonderland, as young women growing up we were often at the mercy of "fun house" rules in terms of the dizzying changes in body images, styles, trends, fashions, mores, rules, messages (both subliminal and overt), dictums, orders, and ultimatums. We've been *Cosmo*'d, *Vogue*'d, *Mademoiselle*'d, *Glamour*'d, and *Seventeen* magazine'd to death. One year the buxom, full-figured blond is everyone's ideal; the next year it's dark, exotic, ethnic beauties; and the year after that it's flat-chested, hollow-cheeked, pre-pubescents. Like Alice, you're torn between one pill that makes you larger and one pill that makes you small. All this attention paid to how you look and so little emphasis on the importance of how you *feel*.

If the sexual hunger I spoke of earlier is as natural to you as your physical appetite, then the only thing that could interfere with its natural expression by your natural Bad Girl self is mental manipulation and conditioning. In the same way that Chinese women had to bind their feet to keep them small and thus desirable to Chinese men, we have been taught to bind the natural size, shape, and potency of our sexual selves! Doesn't that make you angry? Doesn't that seem completely unfair? Doesn't it make you want to rip off the chains that bind you, free yourself from those constraints, and wiggle your toes in the sands of freedom?

Of course it does. *No one* should have the power to cram us into a mold and make us conform to *their* vision of how we should be sexually. Your sexuality should be as free to grow and develop on its own as your feet. Unfortunately, however, that has not been the case.

Well, enough is enough! We know better now! Let the beginning of the end of sexually repressed, unnatural, Good Girl behavior start with all of the brave and powerful women who read this book and learn to unleash the Bad Girl within. We know now that bad is natural, that bad is healthy, and that bad is *better* than good.

From now on, we *reject* anyone else's ideas, opinions, or needs that can't accommodate our experience of ourselves as Bad women— women who were born to be bad and have a right to embrace that. Bad Girls are in control. A Bad Girl doesn't hand over the reins of power to anything or anybody that tries to diminish, belittle, or otherwise shake her faith in herself. Bad Girls *know* that they are fabulous, no matter what. I know you want it, *you* know you want it. So let's get to it, right now.

Shifting into Gear

If I've been doing my job here, I've already described a way of living that must sound pretty darn good. I've probably gotten you more than a little bit excited by the prospect of being truly bad. But now what? How do we take that "pie in the sky" and put it on a plate down here on planet earth?

I'm sure you're familiar with the expression, "You can lead a horse to water but you can't make her drink." In many ways, this old saying holds a powerful truth about the process of change, and about the process of becoming a Bad Girl in particular. I can lead you to the "water," which in this case is a reservoir of sexual feeling, sexual power and sexual passion that *already* exists inside you. *I* am not the water and I can't provide the water for you. I *can*, however, act as a sort of divining rod to help you locate that reservoir within yourself and teach you how to tap into that reservoir so that you have total access.

One way I am going to help you find that reservoir of sexuality is to lead you through a series of exercises. Some of these will be mental exercises and some will be more physical. All of them are designed to help you break through the layers of OPNs (other people's notions) that have grown thick over the years, trapping your Bad Girl in their muck. The tools and skills you'll acquire by doing the exercises will enable you to hear and then speak in your own *true* sexual "voice" (and boy is that voice ever SEXY! You'll see . . .). So grab a knife and fork, because it won't be long before that pie in the sky is within reach, and you're enjoying your first delectable bite.

BUT FIRST, AN IMPORTANT CAUTION

Before we go to the first exercise, I need to take a brief, but very serious time-out right here to address the subject of sexual abuse. If you have been a victim of rape, incest, or any other kind of sexual violence, I would encourage you to consult with a therapist before embarking on any type of sexual self-help program, including this one. Although the exercises in this book are designed to be enlightening and fun, they can also stir up a lot of emotion when abuse has been a factor in a woman's life. If you haven't already engaged a professional therapist or counselor to help you deal with the trauma you have suffered, I hope you will do so; I hate to think of anyone trying to bear the weight of that pain alone.

exercise 1:

Writing Your "Mission Statement"

We're going to start our exercise program by taking a few moments to do something every Bad Girl does: announce your Bad intentions.

- For this exercise, you will need paper and a pen. Since there will be a number of writing exercises in this book, many of a very personal nature, I recommend you use a dedicated notebook (not loose sheets of paper). This notebook and its contents should be "for your eyes only." To do these exercises effectively, it is important that you know your privacy is protected.

You don't need an audience right now—not yet—but there are a few things you do need to start saying to the most important person in your sexual universe: you. Do you remember what I said about a Bad Girl's intentions? *To be hot, to be in touch, and to be fully sexual alive with herself and with her sexual partner.* I want you to write these words in large clear letters on the page in front of you. But make them personal, like this: **"To be hot, to be in touch, and to be fully sexually alive with myself and my sexual partner."** This is your sexual future. It is your personal mission statement. Read it to yourself, then read it out loud. Read it and believe in it. You are already closer than you think.

exercise 2:

Defining Moments in Your Good Girl History

Ever dream about doing a little time-traveling? Here's your chance. This exercise involves going back in time to identify the instances and situations in your life when your sexuality got derailed, shut down, or set aside. It's time to reexamine those defining moments; to discover those forks in the road that steered you away from your authentic sexual self.

Once again, you will need your notebook for this exercise.

- Close your eyes and take several deep breaths. Breathe in through your nose and exhale through your mouth. Take your time—don't rush. You want to be in a relaxed, yet alert state of mind. Silently affirm that your memory will work perfectly and that you will remember everything you need to know.

- Let your mind drift back in time. You're 20, 15, 12. You're in college, high school, grade school. **When is the first time you can remember receiving the message that your sexual thoughts, sexual feelings, and/or sexual behaviors were not okay?** Try not to censor, judge, or comment on yourself. We're just detectives here, looking for clues. When the memory comes to you, **write it down.** Try to be very specific. If it comes in fragments, or was just kind of a feeling that you started to get at a certain time in your life, try to describe it as best you can and write that down, too.

- Now ask yourself: Who did this message come from? How did it make me feel at the time? Did it affect my behavior at the time? If so, how?

- When was the next defining sexual moment? The next? The next? Continue following this timeline of sexual moments up to the present day. There are probably some incidents that are so vivid you don't have to dig for them at all. There may be other memories that are more subtle—a magazine article that you read once, for example, or a casual comment from a teacher or a classmate. Don't discount anything; **if it comes into your mind, write it down.** You can always decide later if it doesn't have any merit.

You may find that you need several sessions to complete this exercise. Some women have so many memories, they can't write them all in one sitting. Other women draw a blank and have to really sit with the question in their minds for a long time before any memories present themselves. There is no right or wrong. You are simply *not* allowed to beat up on yourself in any way during this process—doctor's orders!

Piecing the Puzzle Together

Once you have completed Exercise 2, having excavated as many memories as you can and having committed them to paper, it's time to take a few steps back and look at those memories from your current vantage point. Looking back on those defining moments that you had as you were growing up, how does the distance of time affect the way that you view the incidents *today*? What can you see about these moments now that you couldn't see then? Who was trying to control you? Who was trying to manipulate you? And why did they have a personal agenda that did not support the growth and development of your healthy sexuality?

Do you think you would have the same reaction to each of these messages if you were hearing them for the first time *today*? Probably not. You might laugh at some, get angry at some, and not even notice others. I'm pretty sure that even the most powerful messages wouldn't have the same power over you today, if you were hearing them for the first time, because you're not a little girl/teenager/virgin anymore. You've grown up. You may feel very young at times, particularly when other adults are still trying to control your sexuality, but you're not that same person. In fact, the maturity you've developed since these defining moments first occurred is probably helping you have a pretty compassionate attitude toward the little girl/young woman you just wrote about. She's had to suffer through a lot of other people's ignorance and fear. But can't you see it for what it is now: *other people's ignorance and fear*? So let me ask you another question: **Can you see any reason why you should allow these experiences to continue ruling your sex life?**

It reminds me of a story a sex therapist I trained under used to tell to new clients to demonstrate the power of our earliest lessons:

> *When animal handlers begin working with baby elephants that are being trained for the circus, they drive heavy stakes into the ground to which they tether the baby elephants by a chain (sort of like a dog on a leash) so that they can't run away. The untrained baby elephant strains against the chain at first in its natural rambunctious state, trying to break free. After several weeks though, the elephant stops testing the chain, having learned that its struggle against the restraint is futile. As the animal grows, the handlers continue to "stake" the elephant. Even though the elephant soon grows to a size that would allow it to easily pull the stake from the ground and run free, it has long since stopped trying. The elephant is convinced that the stake is stronger than it is, and has lost the will to even try. Psychologists call this "learned helplessness."*

Many of us are not that different from the baby circus elephants. We are still tethered to the past by old, outdated modes of behavior that were forced upon us when we were young and impressionable—still committed to being "little." We have forgotten that we are big and strong now, with the power to break free of the chains of the past and choose our own destiny. You are big and strong. You can break free from the past. You will be who and what *you* want to be. Say it out loud:

I am big and strong.
I can break free from the past.
I will be who and what *I* want to be.

Make this your battle cry as you progress through this book, if you like. It feels good, doesn't it? If you're starting to feel a little flutter in your chest, that's your Bad Girl doing her warm-ups; your words are music to her ears. Each time you affirm your strength and your right to be who you really are, sexually or otherwise, you give your Bad Girl room to breathe, room to move, room to be.

Is Your Good Girl Doing Anyone Any Good?

When I first started teaching classes in human sexuality, one of my most memorable students was a young woman named Ellen. Ellen was "good to the bone." She always wore her pretty brown hair up in a sensible bun. She wore no makeup, no nail polish, no jewelry except for her wedding band. She had a penchant for puffed sleeves and gingham. I have since stopped being surprised to see women like Ellen in my classroom, but at the time, I have to admit I was mystified. Driven by my desire to know more about her, I decided to ask all of the students what had prompted them to enroll in my class.

Ellen revealed that she was there at the urging of her husband. She admitted that he was anxious to have her learn more about the scope of human sexuality. Apparently, he believed her definitions were unreasonably narrow. Ellen was a virgin when she married. She refused to have sex more than once a week (Saturdays at 9:00 P.M.) She didn't see the need for any kind of sex except intercourse, missionary style.

As the class progressed and the students worked their way through many of the exercises that are also in this book, Ellen's history started coming to light. She was the oldest of three whose mother died when she was eleven years old. Her father kept a tight rein on her, relying on her to cook, clean, and baby-sit. There wasn't a lot of time for playing or being a kid. The more she developed, the more her father's anxiety increased, fueled by his own memories of what he was like as a teenage boy. He would constantly warn Ellen how dangerous boys were and remind her of her responsibilities at home. He would say, "You let a boy touch you and the next thing you know you'll wind up with a baby in your belly." (When he was sixteen, he had actually gotten *his* very first girlfriend pregnant.) "Then what will we do? Only tramps act up to boys. Be a Good Girl, Ellen. Make your mother proud of you."

Ellen's father was desperate to keep her in line because he needed someone to help take care of the house, take care of the other children, and take care of him. He was willing to exaggerate, lie, intimidate and threaten to keep Ellen from exploring her sexual feelings and growing up too fast. I'm not trying to demonize Ellen's father; he wasn't an evil man. He never expected to be raising three children on his own and he did the best he could. It's just that his best wasn't good enough to spare Ellen his draconian methods of child rearing.

As the class progressed, Ellen came to discover that even though she was no longer in her father's house, no longer responsible for her brother and sister, married to a man she loved, and had a college degree and a good job, she was still playing by her father's rules, still dancing to his tune, still being Good for him. Her father's harsh words were still having their desired affect on Ellen: disconnecting her from her sexuality so that she would continue to serve his needs. Once Ellen saw how she had been manipulated, she was able to start accepting an increasing array of sexual feelings, thoughts, and acts as normal and natural. It was a joy and a privilege as her teacher to watch her begin to integrate her growing sexual awareness into her behavior, her language, and her life.

So . . . Who does *YOUR* Good Girl serve? Who are you still doing the dance for? What ghosts from the past are haunting your present sex life? If you are like the overwhelming majority of women I know, your Good Girl is *only* serving ghosts—still taking care of people from your past who don't even care anymore if you're good or bad. Even worse, you are doing yourself a disservice. If there *is* someone in your life who still has an investment in your being a little girl or a Good Girl, you know the time has come to put that person in his or her place, stare that person down, shut that person up. This is your *life* we're talking about. If they want to be good, that's their choice—don't let them make it yours.

Bad Girls Feel Good about Being Bad

Feel the Power

I hope you are beginning to understand how vital it is for you to be Bad, and how necessary it is for you to embrace your Bad Girl self. Let's face it: there is nothing good about being a Good Girl. Being good robs you of your strength. It robs you of your inherent power as an adult, sexual woman with healthy appetites and impulses. It robs you of your authentic self. A Good Girl is, plain and simple, a cheated woman.

When you give up on being bad, you give your partner *all of the power*!

- It's up to **him** *when* you have sex
- It's up to **him** *how* you have sex
- It's up to **him** whether or not you have an orgasm
- It's up to **him** to provide any passion or ardor that may or may not be present when you make love

What, please tell me, is *good* about that? Not one single thing.

If you walk into a dark room, you don't just stand there in the dark until someone else comes along to turn the lights on, do you? No! You feel around on the wall until you find the switch and then *you flip the switch yourself!* I want you to think of this process of reclaiming your Bad Girl in the same way. Being a Good Girl has kept you in the dark for way too long. No more waiting for "the right man" or "the right time" to bring you out of your dark Good Girl prison and into the light. You need to start feeling around for that light switch yourself, find the keys to that prison cell door, and free yourself to step into your sexuality, your strength, and your power. Man or no man, your time has arrived—the time to reclaim your sexual self and feel absolutely *great* about being utterly *bad.*

Welcome to My World

Here we are, almost at the end of just one chapter, and you've already accomplished so much! You have my respect and admiration for taking such a bold step toward your goal of being the fabulous Bad Girl it is your birthright to be. But before we move on to chapter 2, let's take one last opportunity here to remind yourself, and tell the universe, all about your newfound desire to bring in the bad.

exercise 3:

Inviting Your Bad Girl in from the Cold

- Find a mirror in your home that allows you to see your entire body. Face the mirror. The Eskimos have more than 100 words for "snow." You're about to invent more than 100 ways to say "I want to be bad."

- Look into your eyes. *Start talking*:
  "I want to be bad."
  "I am bad. Very bad. Very, very bad."
  "I deserve to be bad."
  "I ache to be bad."
  "I live to be bad."
  "Bad is beautiful."
  "Bad looks good on me."
  "I wear bad well." *Keep going . . .*

Get the picture? Now, I know a lot of you couldn't help giggling at first. That's to be expected. Your Good Girl isn't completely in remission yet, and we'll keep working on that as the book continues. But hopefully as you went along, the phrases became more anchored in you and you were able to say them with increasing conviction. Truth is, if you got just one single phrase out of your mouth—just one—you've already met the biggest challenge. You've punctured the first hole in that good-for-nothing Good Girl persona. It only gets easier from here.

So, where *do* we go from here? We've learned what has kept you from being bad. We've gone to great lengths to see why it's *important* to be bad. We've explored the tyranny of being "good," and we've put some of that "Good Girl" stuff behind us. So much for the past. It's time to step into the future—a future where Good Girls aren't welcome. The time has come, you naughty, naughty girls, to give your undivided attention to learning how to *be* bad.

Chapter 2

Bad Girls Have Sex on the Brain

What are you thinking about this very moment? I hope the answer is SEX. Are you thinking about your lover's mouth on various parts of your body? Are you thinking about the thrill of penetration? Are you thinking about your next orgasm? If you're thinking about flossing your teeth, I'm concerned but not completely discouraged.

Experts tell us that most of us have a sexual thought every sixty seconds. What they don't tell us is what we *do* with those sexual thoughts. Well, I'm going to tell you what most of us do with those thoughts: we push them away. Ask yourself these questions, and be honest with your answers. How often do you let yourself think about sex? And how often do you let yourself get lost in those feelings? Do you let yourself fill with desire on a daily basis, or do you tell yourself that you need to be thinking about other more "important" things, more "responsible" things, more "mature" things? Do you even *have* a sexual thought every sixty seconds, or does it seem more like sixty days?

Here is something you need to remember for the rest of your life: **Bad Girls never stop thinking about sex**. From the time they open their eyes in the morning until they close their eyes at night to sleep, sex is always there. It's there when they watch the morning news ("Mmmm, if I could just get Matt Lauer alone in a room for half an hour . . .") and when they read the morning paper ("God bless Jockey and Calvin Klein . . ."). They have sexual fantasies on the way to work. At work. And on the way home. They think about it over dinner. They see it in their dreams. Morning, noon, and night, sex is always a part of their world.

Too many women have the very bad habit of compartmentalizing sex. We tell ourselves, "there's a time and place for everything," instead of letting ourselves embrace and enjoy the flood of sexuality that could be with us every hour of the day. Thinking about sex does not interfere with your driving, your shopping, or your ability to work. Thinking about sex *enhances* everything. It keeps you feeling fully alive. It keeps you ready for sex at a moment's notice. It also sends a telepathic message to your partner (or intended partner) that puts him on notice, too. It puts him on edge. It puts him on pins and needles. It puts him where you want him, and keeps him there . . . waiting for you. That is what you want, isn't it?

Four Types of Women, Four Ways to Think about Sex

You know that there are different blood types (type A, type O, type B, etc.), and that there are different skin types (combination, oily, dry), but did you know that there are different *sexual* types, and that each of these sexual types has a very different way of *thinking* about sex? Just as it is important to know your blood or skin type in order to effectively treat a condition you may have, it's imperative to know what *sexual* type you are for the very same reason.

After many years of observation and study, it has become clear to me that there are basically only four different sexual categories that women fall under. Which one sounds most like you?

The Bad Girl

Let's start with the namesake of this book. A Bad Girl is completely at ease and accepting of all the various facets of her sexual personality. She knows what she likes, how she likes it, and who she likes it with. She is so in control of herself and so clear about her sexual boundaries that she is *free* to be completely wild within that context (Don't understand that statement? You will by the end of the book. Keep reading!) A Bad Girl's sexuality is her crowning glory. In fact, a Bad Girl wears her sexuality as naturally and as shamelessly as a head of flowing, shiny, healthy hair. She is, as I said earlier, *always* thinking about sex, and it shows in the most positive ways.

A Bad Girl is so at ease with her erotic self that her sexuality is exciting for others to see, beautiful to behold, and makes men yearn to touch it—just like a beautiful head of hair. She has probably worked hard to achieve the relationship she has with her sexuality and she isn't thrown when it makes someone uncomfortable or someone has a problem with it. She is no one's slave and no one's servant (unless they're playing a game!). She is true to herself; first and foremost.

Frankly, I doubt there are going to be too many Bad Girls reading this book. Why would they? Bad Girls know they're bad; they've already got it. They're more likely to be reading *Discover Your Sensual Potential* or *How to Make Love All Night*! Also, Bad Girls are in the minority to begin with. If there are a hundred women in a room, it is probably safe to say that no more than ten of them are really Bad.

The Librarian

The Librarian is the polar opposite of the Bad Girl—a woman who makes it her full time job to *not* think about sex. I'm sorry to be using such an obvious stereotype for my label (and I apologize to all of those women who may be toiling over the card catalogs while boiling over with sexuality), but I know that the image is one that we can all immediately conjure in our mind's eye. The Librarian is shut as tight as an obscure botany textbook wedged between a bunch of research periodicals in the Reserved section of the library. This sexual type is more than just a bit shut down. The Librarian has constructed a personality and a life that is completely devoid of sexual excitement. Even when she is having sex—which isn't very often—she isn't feeling very *sexual*. It is, after all, hard to feel very sexual in the library—especially when you can't make any noise!

Like the Bad Girls, there will probably only be a select few of these sexual celibates (you don't have to *be* celibate to *feel* celibate) who pick up this book. However, the reason they won't be reading the book is entirely different than the Bad Girls' reason. If a Bad Girl is *committed* to enjoying, fostering, and exploring her sexual passion and power, a Librarian is equally *committed* to protecting, ignoring, and denying her sexual truth. These women are even harder to find than the Bad Girls; out of a hundred women in a room, I would expect to see only a handful of Librarians.

Of the four different sexual types, I have the deepest sympathy for the Librarians. Something in their lives has simply made the prospect of a sexual identity, of sexual pleasure and enjoyment, too risky. Often the Librarian sublimates her sexuality by living for (and in) her work. She may be very accomplished, but she just can't let herself think about sex. She needs to do everything possible to make that world disappear.

If you see yourself in this description and you're still reading this book, *congratulations!* Something is obviously shifting for you. But I expect the number of Librarians reading this book to be very small.

So far, my sexual type-casting has accounted for less than 20 percent of the female population at large. What about everyone else? The next two sexual types comprise the remaining 80 percent or more of the female population—the majority of women on this perfect planet of ours. So prepare to be hit closer to home!

The Closet Cleopatra

The Closet Cleo is the sexiest woman alive . . . late at night, alone, in her deepest, darkest fantasies, that is. This is the soccer mom next door, your dental hygienist, and very possibly, *you*.

Outwardly, if you're a Cleo, you're chipper, sunny, energetic; a bit "speeded up," most likely. You dress nicely: Eddie Bauer, the Gap, Talbots; you've probably been dressing the same basic way since high school. You care about your appearance and probably err on the side of caution when it comes to wardrobe (wouldn't want to show too much skin!). But this is the same woman who really, really wants to have one of those sexy boudoir photos taken (if she hasn't already); even if she does only hang it in her closet (where she keeps *all* her sexual secrets).

This is a woman who can have a fantasy of making love on a bearskin rug in front of a roaring fire, but if actually given the opportunity, would demurely decline with, "No, it's too hot!" or "No, it's too cold!" or "No, I couldn't do that to the bear!" In Closet Cleo's *interior* life, she's familiar with sexual desire, sexual scenarios, and sexy behavior. But in the real world, well, that's another story. In the real world, Closet Cleo finds all sorts of reasons why she **can't**.

- She **can't** wear that skimpy negligee (because the kids could come in, she'll look ridiculous, it's "uncomfortable," etc.)
- She **can't** say "those words" (what if somebody overheard?)
- She **can't** do "that" (because only you-know-who's and you-know-what's do "that")

So what is Closet Cleo's problem? Closet Cleo is not letting herself get fully hooked up to her interior sexual life. She has banished the woman she dreams of being to an indeterminate time-out, left to sit in the corner, staring at the wall, living for the rare times when she gets to make a brief appearance.

Does Cleo think about sex? You bet she does. She thinks about sex a lot, but she isn't comfortable with most of those thoughts, so she hides them or dismisses them or quickly censors them. She is her own worst sexual critic.

Closet Cleos can see it, feel it, and dream it, but they have a problem doing it, living it, and being it. So near yet so far. That's a feeling I know so well, because if I had to describe my own sexual type before I embraced my Bad Girl self, Closet Cleo would have been it. I was not alone. I believe that Cleos make up the largest chunk of the female population. Of those one hundred women in the room, I would estimate that more than sixty of them are Cleos.

Ms. Christmas Tree

I have a lot of affection for the fourth and final sexual type we're going to take a look at. I call her Ms. Christmas Tree because she tends to be lit up like one. Ms. Tree also thinks about sex a lot, but she thinks about it in a very different way than a Bad Girl or a Cleo.

This is a woman for whom the term "less is more" makes absolutely no sense. To her, less is just . . . less. If she's wearing a short skirt, then she also has to wear a push-up bra, thigh-high boots, big hair, and lots of jewelry. Ms. Tree wears her sexuality on her sleeve. She *looks* like she's really into sex. She *looks* like she's really comfortable with her sexuality. She *looks* like she has a lot of sexual confidence. But as we all know, looks can be deceiving. Ms. Tree is doing everything she can to convince the outside world and *herself* that she is hot, hot, hot, but Ms. Tree's sad little secret is that she's not, not, not. Inside, where it counts most, Ms. Tree doesn't feel much of anything.

This can be a little confusing to some of you Cleos (and Librarians, too). When a Cleo looks at a Christmas Tree, she isn't sure what to think. One voice is saying, "Something is wrong with this picture," but another voice is wondering, "Maybe she knows something I don't know," or "Maybe she has something I don't have." It's easy to understand how Ms. Tree can get you confused. After all, there is a lot of sex in the presentation—there just isn't a lot of *sexuality*.

I will never forget the first time a Ms. Tree, who was taking my human sexuality class, came to my office and poured her heart out to me. We had been discussing orgasms in class the hour before and I had noticed that she had remained unusually quiet. Too ashamed to admit it in front of her classmates, Ms. Tree tearfully confessed to me in private that she had *never had an orgasm*; neither through masturbation nor with a partner. It was everything I could do to maintain my professional demeanor. I mean, the young woman sitting in front of me *looked* like she was born to be wild, a real hot number. But here she was, telling me that she didn't get what all the fuss over sex was about because in her experience, sex had never amounted to much.

I was amazed. But every semester there is at least one Ms. Tree who comes to me with the same admission, and I know there are a lot more Ms. Trees in my classes who are suffering in silence with the same problem.

So what *is* her problem? Ms. Tree is just going through the motions. Her interior landscape is as barren as her exterior is lavishly adorned. The lights are on but nobody's home. Because Ms. Tree doesn't have a sexual compass to guide her, she is constantly overcompensating by trying to be all things to all people. She is trying to give men the presentation she thinks they want, trying to give women the presentation she thinks they envy. That's a lot of work for very little reward.

Ms. Tree wants to feel Bad and look Bad and *be* Bad but she doesn't know how to get there. She is always looking to the outside for cues and clues, but she keeps missing the boat because she still doesn't understand that being Bad starts on the inside from your sexual center.

Ms. Tree needs to move into her house. She needs to learn to inhabit her own body. She has some idea of what sexy *looks* like (although she tends to overdo it), but she has very little idea of how "sexy" might actually *feel*. Like Closet Cleo, Ms. Christmas Tree has to learn to *slow down* and allow her feelings and desires time to surface into her conscious mind.

It all starts with the way you think about sex.

How many Ms. Trees are there out there? In that room of a hundred women, maybe fifteen or twenty.

So there you have it. Four different women, four different sexual types, and four different ways to think about sex. Ready to ask yourself the big question: Which type sounds like you? Keep in mind that I have painted a rather extreme picture of Closet Cleo, Ms. Tree, and our Librarian so that the traits of each type would be clear to you. Most women aren't walking caricatures, but will find that their behavior does place them more in one category than another.

So now you've defined yourself and your sexual type. You've put a name and a set of descriptions to your appearance, attitude, and behavior. Is it a relief? A surprise? A little of both? What does it tell you about the way you think about sex? *Now* what do you do?

Laying the Foundation

The purpose of defining your sexual type is to know what it is we're dealing with; what we're up against, so to speak. Since I'm certain that that the Librarians haven't taken this book off the shelf yet, that the genuine Bad Girls are out living their Bad Girl lives, and that I am talking to an audience of Closet Cleos and Ms. Christmas Trees here, let me summarize accordingly.

If you're a *Closet Cleo* you now know that:

- You deny your sexual thoughts.
- You tend to squelch your sexual expression.
- You're stuck at an earlier point in your sexual development.

If you're a *Ms. Tree* you now know that:

- It's time to cultivate your sexual landscape.
- Sexy starts inside, *then* expresses outwardly (not the other way around).
- It's time to learn what turns *you* on!

The symptoms experienced by Cleo and Ms. Tree are different, but the cure is the same, and that cure starts with a painless injection of **sexual thought.** If you can't think about sex with complete comfort, if you can't think about sex without any judgment, if you can't think about sex without worrying about his sexual needs, you're on a treadmill that will never take you to the Bad side of town. Sexual thought needs to become an integrated factor in your waking life. Sexual thought is literally the *foundation* from which your Bad Girl will spring. Sexual thought is the Bad Girl's best friend.

Planting the Seeds of Sexual Thought

I have always loved art, but I never thought that it was something that had the power to affect my life on a daily basis. Well, I was wrong. Several years ago, I went with a friend to a summer art fair in Los Angeles and wound up making a purchase that changed my sexual landscape, both external and internal. Frankly, it changed my life.

My friend and I were meandering through the aisles at the fair, pausing briefly here and there to look at the many beautiful drawings, paintings, and sculptures, when suddenly, out of the corner of my eye, I glimpsed something gleaming in the sun just across the way. I threaded my way through all of the bodies and finally found myself standing before it. It was, to my eye, the most beautiful sculpture I had ever seen.

Bad Girls Have Sex on the Brain

The sculpture is called *Extase* (pronounced "ecstasy"), and it is a white Italian marble statue of a beautiful nude. The woman is seated in a modified splits, except her front leg is bent back beneath her at the knee. Her right arm is fully extended behind her and rests gracefully on her outstretched leg. Her back is arched with desire to the point that her hair is hanging straight down and she is looking toward the sky. Her left arm is raised and bent at the elbow; the edge of her palm rests languidly against her cheek. Her entire body is one sleek, sexy, curvaceous line. She is the very essence of female sexuality.

You may be wondering why I'm sharing this very personal aspect of my life with you. I'll tell you why. *Extase* is the first thing I see when I come home every day and open my front door. I may have just spent an hour in bumper-to-bumper traffic, I may have a whole evening's worth of work ahead of me, I may have dropped the bag of groceries that had the eggs in it on my slate floor—all of that may be true. But when I lay eyes on that sculpture, all of that falls away and I am *immediately* put back in touch with the *me who I want to be:* the *slow* me, the *feeling* me, the *sexual* me. I *see* myself in that sculpture. The state of ecstasy so perfectly captured in this sculpture is the state I aspire to integrate ever more fully into my daily life. I see my best self in that sculpture.

The sculpture helps *plant the seed* of sexual thought in my brain whenever I see it (which is quite often!). It is, for me, a *sexual totem*. One of the definitions of the word "totem," as given in the dictionary, is: "Something that serves as an emblem or revered symbol." My sculpture is both an emblem and a revered symbol of my sexuality and my *connection* to it. This totem reconnects me to my sexual core.

Once I was a skeptic (and even a cynic), but now I am a true believer in a totem's power to transform a woman's relationship to her sexuality. There is something *magical* about having something *tangible* in your personal environment, something you can see and touch. The act of declaring, *"This is what is sexual to me,"* frees and empowers you. Placing your Sexual Totem in a conspicuous place is a clear message to *yourself* that you're not ashamed to be sexual.

Finding Your Totem

I went for far too many years before I discovered that a sexual totem could enrich my life to such a great extent. Today, I make it a point of

33

suggesting to the women I teach and to the women who read my books that they find a sexual totem and place it in a prominent place in their homes.

What will it be? Will it be a sensual photograph? An erotic drawing? A painting? A poster? A sculpture that captures *your* sexual essence? When choosing your totem:

- Make sure you can see it without having to open any-thing (like a box or a book) or having to dig it out from under a pile of stuff. You want it *in* your environment.
- You should be able to easily place yourself in the scene depicted by the totem. You don't want to feel like you're on the outside looking in.
- Your totem can be very abstract or very concrete—the important thing is that it feels very sexual to you.
- Try to place the totem in a conspicuous place in your home that you pass by regularly. You want to be able to see your totem frequently so that it can work its magic as often as possible. You don't have to explain it to anyone—you just need to display it.
- Don't choose something that embarrasses you. Your totem should be a source of pride, not a source of embarrassment or shame.

Saying Goodbye to Good Girl Totems

Have you found that special object that is going to light up your Bad Girl life? That's great, but you're not quite finished. There is a "part B" to this totem ritual, and it involves a little "closet cleaning."

If you look around your home, I'll bet you will come across some-thing that was given to you when you were a young girl that instantly reminds you of your girlhood. For me, it's a Lladro sculpture of a little girl holding a basket of flowers that my mother gave to me many years ago. For you, it could be something like a music box, a photo, or a stuffed animal. You may not realize it, but that object acts as a sexual totem too. Instead of connecting you to your most adult, sexual self, it connects you to your least adult, most chaste, Good Girl self. Take a good look around because I know it's there somewhere, staring at you.

Bad Girls Have Sex on the Brain

It was probably given to you by a parent, grandparent, or someone else equally libido-dampening! Have you found it? Now brace yourself. Because . . .

it has to go.

You don't need to throw it away—especially if it has sentimental value (or, even better, dollar value—*Antiques Road Show*, here we come!). But *please*, put it out of sight. You may be so used to looking at this Good Girl totem that you don't even really see it any more. But just because it has become a part of the scenery doesn't mean that it doesn't have an effect on you. Believe me, it does, and your *new* Bad Girl sexual totem needs to be able to do its work unimpeded by the mixed message of your asexual girlhood totem.

So take a real good look around your personal environment and try to find the item (or items) that tie you tightly to your "little girl" self. It's time to put those things aside and replace them with items that are more age-appropriate, more sexually appropriate, more Bad Girl appropriate. If you want to be a Bad Girl, you're going to have to do a little bit of growing up. And that process starts with the messages you welcome into your head. Good Girl symbols goodbye, Bad Girl symbols *hel-lo!*

Bad Girls Have a One-Track Mind

A Bad Girl can find something sexy in just about *anything*. The reason for this is that her sexuality is the organizing *context* for her thoughts. She has successfully developed a one-track mind, and I say that with kudos. Just as pessimists can find something negative in every occurrence, and optimists can find something positive, Bad Girls can find something *sexual* in virtually every object, person, and situation that presents itself. Do you have any idea how much *fun* that is? It doesn't mean that she feels compelled to act on what she sees, thinks, or feels, by any stretch of the imagination. But as you might imagine, Bad Girls are never bored!

Let me illustrate for you exactly how that translates into an average day in the life of your typical Bad Girl, and compare it to the typical Good Girl experience.

The Good Girl's Guide to Bad Girl Sex

The Morning Shower

Bad Girl: Thinks of her morning shower as the perfect opportunity to connect to her body and wake the senses. She uses a luxurious, aromatic shower gel and takes the opportunity to self-massage, awaken her erotic senses, and perhaps even bring herself to orgasm, if time allows.

Good Girl: Thinks of her morning shower as her morning shower. Scrubs herself clean with the same brand of bar soap her mother bought for her when she was a kid. Doesn't see, feel, or enjoy her body.

The Elevator Ride to Her Floor at Work

Bad Girl: Thinks of the ride to her floor as a chance to do some erotic window-shopping. She spots a pair of great buns in the crush of bodies in front of her (and not on the coffee wagon!) and immediately begins to fantasize about what it would feel like to give them a firm squeeze. A Mona Lisa smile plays provocatively along her lips.

Good Girl: Thinks of the ride to her floor as an oppressive five minutes she must grin and bear. She spots the sweet cheeks in the gabardines too, but immediately averts her eyes, suddenly finding the lighted display of numbers over the elevator door absolutely riveting. Almost by rote, she then starts ticking off all the items on her daily "to-do" list.

Lunch

Bad Girl: Thinks of mealtime as a sensual experience. She goes to her favorite Italian restaurant and orders a plate of linguini with olive oil. She chews each bite slowly and thoroughly, enjoying the tastes and texture of each mouthful. She doesn't rush through the meal; she knows she *deserves* to take her time.

Good Girl: Thinks of food as fuel. She stays at her desk working through most of her lunch hour and then grabs a cold sandwich from the vending machine in the company lunchroom. She wolfs down the sandwich standing up. With a knot in her stomach, she rushes back to her desk.

Bad Girls Have Sex on the Brain

The Afternoon Staff Meeting

Bad Girl: Okay, she's not looking forward to this any more than the Good Girl is, but she keeps an open mind. Today it pays off when she notices how much her boss's hands look like the hands of her lover. Suddenly, she's remembering last night and just how busy those hands of her lover were. A ho-hum staff meeting becomes a lot more interesting and she finds herself able to pay close attention.

Good Girl: Thinks of every staff meeting as an unbearable chore. She feels herself being lulled into a state of near unconsciousness by her boss's monotonous tone of voice. She's caught off guard when her boss asks her a question and is embarrassed when she has to ask him to repeat it.

The Friday Evening Commute Home

Bad Girl: Thinks of the drive home as her time alone to relax, let go of the day, and fantasize about the evening ahead. She finds music to suit her mood (she keeps dozens of her favorite CDs in the car) and by the time she reaches her front door she has let go of the day's challenges and is ready to embrace the evening and its (hopefully) sensual surprises.

Good Girl: Thinks of the drive home as the absolute worst part of the day. She gets completely stressed out by the traffic, the bad news on AM radio, and the fresh memory of her embarrassing moment in today's meeting.

Friday Night

Bad Girl: She has, in so many ways (both directly and indirectly), been thinking about and preparing for this evening all day long. Now she is primed, pumped, and ready. It may not be an all-night sexual marathon (after all, she *is* tired), but having sex with her partner tonight is the natural culmination of all she has put into her day.

Good Girl: Can't stop thinking about the day, her job, and all of the errands she needs to run tomorrow. She only has sex because her partner wants to. She cannot shift gears enough to connect to her erotic core. She falls asleep wishing that things were different.

37

Am I exaggerating here? Maybe a little. Being bad isn't always an every-single-minute-of-the-day experience, but it can come close on some days, particularly as the end of the work week approaches.

When you contrast the Good Girl experience with the Bad Girl experience, putting them side by side, it's pretty obvious who's having more fun moment by moment and getting more out of life, isn't it? So what's a Good Girl to do? How exactly **do** you make the transition? If your day sounds a lot more like the GG's than the BG's, what's the fastest, easiest, and most effective way to start flooding your mind with sex, sex, and more sex? It starts by waking up each morning and focusing your attention on the Bad Girl's very best friend.

Meet the Bad Girl's Best Friend

It's 6 A.M. and the shrill buzz of your alarm clock fills the room. You need two more hours of sleep. You need coffee. You need a vacation. How are you going to start thinking about *sex*? Instead of dragging yourself out of bed like you do every morning and forcing yourself to greet the day, you need to take sixty seconds—*just sixty seconds*—to spend time with the Bad Girl's best friend.

Every Bad Girl spends quality time every single day with the Bad Girl's best friend. It's part of her wake-up call, her afternoon break, and her evening nightcap. It gets her going at the crack of dawn and keeps her strong and sexually focused into the wee hours. It's responsible for improving more sex lives than raw oysters, Spanish fly and Victoria's Secret combined. You already have it, and the more time you give it, the more it gives back. It's not a vibrator and it's not your lover's penis, though you want to have those two friends around as much as possible too! What is it?

The Bad Girl's best friend is a muscle; or more accurately, a group of muscles. You may not be familiar with this muscle group now, but you're about to fall in love with it. It's your love muscle, your sex muscle, your "do it to me before I explode" muscle. And it is called, simply, your **PC muscle**.

The pubococcygeal muscle group (PC for short), is the muscle group that supports your pelvic cavity. When it is strong and well-toned, it runs like a taut bridge from your pubis to your tail-bone. This muscle group has a very complex job description—it is one very busy group of muscles—but right now there's one basic piece of information about this muscle you need to know:

> *It has been confirmed that the ability to have an orgasm, and the intensity of that orgasm, correlates with the contraction strength of the PC muscle. Women who don't have orgasms, or who have disappointing "boregasms" tend to have weak PC muscles.*

The math on this is very simple (and perhaps you've started doing it already because I *know* you have a dirty mind): the stronger the PC muscle, the easier, the more frequent, and the more intense the orgasms. *This is something you can control.* And that means that your PC muscle is your ticket to Bad Girl paradise.

Pump It Up!

I bet you've never been more motivated to exercise! The good news is that the PC muscle exercises, which are commonly known as Kegel exercises, or Kegels, for short, are very easy to do. You can do them anytime, anywhere. If you don't already know these exercises, it takes no time at all to learn them. First, you need to locate the PC muscle group precisely to insure that you're burning all your workout calories in the right place.

If you have never done any Kegel exercises, or if you aren't really sure you've ever done them correctly, the first thing you need to do is make sure you know which muscles we are talking about here. This is one of the simplest ways to do that:

- Wait until you have to urinate.
- Sit on the toilet and spread your legs a comfortable distance apart.
- As the urine flow begins, try squeezing off the flow. **The muscle that stops the flow of urine is the PC muscle.**
- Hold for one second. Release.
- Repeat the sequence three more times: hold, release, hold, release, hold, release. If you're squeezing the

right muscle, it should halt the flow each time. Be certain to keep your stomach muscles, thigh muscles, and buttocks muscles completely relaxed. After the last release, empty your bladder completely.

• To really get a feeling for the muscle, insert a finger into your vagina and give it a couple of squeezes.

Some of you may find that you can't completely stop the flow. Not to worry. If you haven't been working the muscle it is probably not very strong, but the PC muscle responds quickly with consistent exercise. Not only will you soon be able to stop your urine flow, but, far more important, *"If you build it, you will come!"* (harder, faster and more often!).

The beauty of Kegel exercises is that you can do them absolutely anywhere: driving, shopping, reading, cooking, or watching TV. And no matter where you are or what else you are doing, within moments you are thinking about sex! So here's your regular workout regimen:

Kegel Exercise #1: Start with a deep, relaxing breath. **Squeeze and hold** the PC muscle for three seconds (counting: one thousand, two thousand, three thousand). Release the muscle completely. Squeeze again. Start with ten squeezes, three times a day. Over the next few weeks, slowly increase the number of squeezes until you can comfortably do twenty-five squeezes per set. If you overdo it and become sore, give the muscle a rest for a few days. Remember, easy does it!

Kegel Exercise #2: *Rapidly* **flex and release** the PC muscle for sets of ten. Start with one set, then, after a week, try to work your way up to two or three sets. This exercise is a little harder to master and should only be attempted after you've been doing the squeezes in Kegel Exercise #1 for several weeks. Otherwise, it's easy to wear yourself out.

Kegel Exercise #3: Maximally contract and *hold* the PC muscle for a full count of ten seconds. At the end of the count, give one quick, deep squeeze and then release. Relax for ten seconds, then repeat for as many times as you *comfortably* can. More is not always better—especially not in the beginning when you're building PC strength for the first time.

Bad Girls Have Sex on the Brain

Sexy Is as Sexy Thinks

I *love* Kegel exercises for so many reasons. They've helped non-orgasmic women become orgasmic, they've helped orgasmic women become more orgasmic, and they've helped many women experience their first *multiple* orgasms (we'll talk about that later!). But that's not all. Women who do Kegels have an easier time during childbirth, and a strong PC muscle contributes to an overall picture of vaginal health, preventing leakage from the bladder when you sneeze or cough, and incontinence in later life. That's a lot of reasons to love Kegels.

But here is why I love Kegels most: On a day to day basis, doing my Kegels keeps me in touch with my womanhood, my sexuality, my *heat*. Doing my Kegels puts me in the mood. Doing my Kegels primes my pump, whets my appetite, and warms me up—they are constant reminders to me that I am a sexual creature and 100 percent w-o-m-a-n. Kegels can do the same for you. That is why these exercises are a key ingredient in the Bad Girl's daily regimen. Doing your Kegels throughout the day will put sex where it belongs: *on your brain*. And when you've got sex on the brain, you are on your way to being completely, utterly BAD.

Not for Women Only

Oh, by the way, your lover has a PC muscle, too! He can strengthen his "love muscle" the very same way. The benefits for him? Firmer erections, delayed ejaculations, stronger orgasms, and stronger ejaculations. If either of you would like to know more about it, I go into detail about the male PC muscle in my book, *How to Make Love All Night*.

The More You Start Thinking about Sex, The More You Keep Thinking about Sex

I have a friend who is an economics professor and a part-time financial planner. Twice a year he gives a free four-day seminar on "prosperity" and twice a year, guess what happens? His income shoots up! The first time he told me this, I laughed. I teased him, "Are you sure that seminar is free?" But you know what? Something very similar has been happening in my life since I first started writing books about sex. Every time I sit down to write a new book and really let my mind immerse itself in the material, my sex life gets better!

You might think that because I have a Ph.D., because I'm a sex therapist, because I teach classes in human sexuality, and because I am a total Bad Girl, that I am always at my sexual peak and immune to any down time. I'd like to say that this is true, but it simply is not. My sex life ebbs and flows for a lot of different reasons. For one thing, being in an academic environment can take a lot of the sexuality out of sex. When I'm teaching classes in human sexuality, I'm thinking a lot more about lesson plans, term papers, and grades than I am about being sexual. When I'm working at the clinic, I am focusing on *other people's* sexual needs, not my own—in fact, I need to keep my personal needs as far away from work as possible.

But man, does that change when I start focusing on a new book. When I start writing, I have only the very best sex on the brain. I start thinking about my own needs and about the very best moments of my own sexual history, and I let myself really get lost in the subject. And that gets very exciting!

In becoming our fullest, most sexual selves, we *all* have blocks, challenges and distractions. In my case, sometimes I can't see the forest for the trees! I get so busy treating sex as a subject, I forget to practice what I preach. But all of that changes when I start thinking hard about the best kind of sex. Not thinking about sex as an academic pursuit, or sex as a problem that requires therapy, or sex as a fascinating subject for research. Just thinking about the gorgeous experience of full-tilt-boogie Bad Girl sex.

I may hold a black belt in Bad Girl sex but that doesn't mean there isn't room for improvement. For me, that improvement starts the moment I release from the outside world and *really* let myself start to think about sex. What will it mean for you? It's going to start with your morning Kegels—your sixty-second Bad Girl wake-up call. It's going to continue as you let go of your Closet Cleo or Christmas Tree thinking and start looking at the world all hours of the day and night through a very different sexual filter. You're going to need to fully embrace your new sexual totem. But for you, all of this is just the beginning. In the chapters that follow, I will teach you many more ways to think, and think hard, about the very best kind of sex. So do one last set of squeezes to refocus that Bad Girl energy, give your new totem a nod, and then turn the page and let's shift into a higher gear.

42

Chapter 3

Bad Girls Dress the Part

Sandy is tired of being a Good Girl. More than anything, she wants to be bad. Every night when Sandy goes to bed she wishes that her lover would grab her and ravage her the way he did when they were first dating. She wishes he would tear her clothes off and make love to her like mad until they both explode. So why, you might ask, does Sandy dress for bed wearing a full-length flannel nightgown that her grandmother gave her for Christmas and a pair of large fuzzy slippers with floppy cloth ears?

Sandy's problem is not a problem with wanting: She knows exactly what she wants. Sandy's problem is that she doesn't look the part. She thinks Bad Girl, but she always looks too "good little girl." The mixture of her messages confuses her partner, particularly since the message of desire is the one that usually stays hidden under the surface.

Some women just don't know how to dress for sex. I'm sure this doesn't surprise you. But here's something that will: The rest of us tend to get this "dressing for sex" thing completely *backwards*. In the beginning of a relationship we go out of our way to look really hot. We buy sexy new underwear and slinky new nighties. We give microscopic attention to the cut of our skirts, the length of our hems, the sheen of our pantyhose, the enticing effect of our panty-line and the number of buttons we leave open on our blouse. It's all very exciting. But truth be told, we are exhausting ourselves in these details during a time when they matter the *least*. Let's face it: in the beginning of a relationship, the sexual tension is so intense that it almost doesn't matter *what* you are wearing or not wearing. Your partner wants you bad, and your clothes come off as quickly as they are put on. It is *later*—as the weeks, the months, and (yes, it does happen!) the years go by, when the tension has lost its dramatic edge—that your clothes really count. This is when your attention to detail sends the kinds of sexual messages both your partner and you really need to hear. This is when your attention to detail creates the kind of sexual tension you are hoping for.

What are your clothes telling your partner about your sexual desire? How do you dress on the days you feel sexy? How do you dress for special dates? How do you dress when you are ready for bed, but not ready for sleep?

When you're in the mood to be Bad, you need to look the part—you need to *look* as bad as you feel. You can't expect a man—not even a man you've known for a very long time—to read your mind like a psychic and know exactly how you feel and what you want right now. You need to send some messages he knows how to read; clear external messages that say, "I'm Bad." Then let those external messages work their way from the outside in, to reach him where he is vulnerable. At the same time, those messages will be working on *you*—giving you permission to *feel* as sexy as you look.

In this chapter, I'm going to help you look your baddest with a little assistance from some invaluable daytime and evening props. We'll talk about necklines, hemlines, shoulders, belly buttons, and the pluses and minuses of baring a lot of skin. We'll talk about panties, bras, stockings, shoes, silk, satin, and soft cotton. We'll even talk about makeup, jewelry, and the impact of hair.

Get ready to say good-bye to your fuzzy flannels, your knee-length shorts, and your politically correct underwear. The goal here is a complete erotic makeover that guarantees results. This is not about dressing like a stripper, a hooker, or an "easy lay." This is about dressing like a woman who knows who she is, knows what she needs, knows what she has to offer, and knows how to send a clear message.

44

Baby, You Can Drive Your Car

If you've ever taken a road trip and hit a long stretch of highway that's taken you through sparsely populated country, you've probably used the cruise control feature that allows you to take your foot off the gas and just steer the car. With the cruise control feature activated, you don't have to pay as much attention to what you're doing. The car drives at one consistent, non-varying speed. You're on autopilot; just rolling along without much thought or effort. Cruise control can be very restful, but it can also be dangerous. It demands so little of you, you can easily fall asleep at the wheel and find yourself in a ditch!

Is your wardrobe on autopilot? When is the last time you took the cruise control off when it comes to how you dress? How many of you are so stuck in a rut clothing-wise, it's as though you have driven into that proverbial ditch and there's nary a tow truck in sight? There's a strong possibility that you are stuck in a kind of wardrobe timewarp; you put the cruise control on sometime back in the '80s or early '90s and haven't really thought about dressing since! They say that women don't even reach their sexual peak until their 40s, but is your wardrobe keeping pace with your increasing maturity and sexuality? Or are you still twenty-one and holding?

Please don't take offense. I don't mean to imply that you haven't added any new pieces or that you are hopelessly out of style, but are you dressing as a cute, stylish girl, or as a sexy, stylish *WOMAN?*

How did you dress in high school? What about in college? Were you Miss Collegiate? Did you sport a chin length bob? Were you really clean-cut, all-American with a rainbow assortment of Polo shirts in your closet? Were you a wild child who wore her hair massively teased out, had more holes than fabric in your jeans, and used safety pins to strategically hold together your Def Leppard T-shirt?

Whether you were the poster child for the preppy look, or you were a quintessential rock and roll chick, how far have you really come in your style of dress? How much have you really changed?

You know your Aunt Minnie? The one who still wears her hair in the beehive? Well, take a good look and be warned, because Aunt Minnie got stuck somewhere in her history, too! Oooh. I know that one hurt a little, and I'm sorry to be so blunt. But sometimes you've got to be cruel to be kind, and if I don't ask the tough questions, who will? You've employed me to help you be Bad, and I take my responsibility seriously!

We talked about clothing a little bit in the previous chapter and where Closet Cleos and Ms. Christmas Trees might be stuck in their wardrobe development. But now we're going to get down and dirty; we're going to go over what you wear and how you wear it with a fine-toothed comb. Your cruise control is about to be disengaged.

Let's Talk About . . .

There is one area that will give your Bad Girl a big boost and have a *huge* impact on your psyche. It's relatively low-cost with a surprisingly high return. It's a change I encourage you to make ASAP, 100 percent, completely, and overnight. Wanna know what it is? It's the stuff *he* can't even see 99 percent of the time and you tend to take for granted: Your *underwear!* Bras, panties, demi and full slips, pantyhose, stockings, camisoles, etc. Lingerie can make or break a Bad Girl. Instead of starting at the top, we're going to start at the bottom. Because it's at the bottom, underneath the many layers you put on and take off on any given day, where the foundation of Badness begins. Picture this:

> *You've been dating a man for several weeks and the sexual tension has been building toward a fever pitch. One morning, before you leave for work, he calls you "spontaneously" and asks you to meet him for dinner at a restaurant in one of the upscale hotels in the city to celebrate the one-month anniversary of the day you met. He remembered! Of course, you say yes. After a totally romantic dinner, your guy surprises you with the news that he has reserved a room for the two of you upstairs. You're so excited you feel like your heart might pound right out of your chest.*
>
> *You go up to the room to find a bowl of luscious, long-stemmed strawberries, real whipped cream, and champagne on ice. There is soft music playing in the background and the lights of the city are twinkling in the distance. Your lover turns down the bed and then turns to you. He slowly begins to disrobe you. He takes his time with each button and kisses every new inch of flesh. He finally gets to the last button of your silk blouse and gently pushes it off your shoulders to*

*expose . . . gak! Your old faded and worn cotton Minnie
Mouse bra you threw on this morning because it was the only
clean bra you had.*

*But your lover is a trooper. Yes, he was definitely thrown
by the Minnie Mouse bra, but he soldiers on. He reaches
around behind you and while holding you in his embrace, he
artfully unzips your skirt. Down to the floor it goes, allowing
him to feast his eyes on . . . oof! Not the enormous "grandma
drawers" with the unraveling waistband?! At this point you'd
like to take some of that whipped cream and cover his eyes
with it, because you are absolutely dying of embarrassment.*

Has this ever happened to you? It reminds me of that great line in
the movie *Jerry Maguire* when the older sister advises the younger sib-
ling not to shave her legs so she won't be tempted to sleep with Jerry
Maguire on their first date! Unless you were born and raised in Europe,
unshaven legs and unshaven armpits are usually a subliminal message
to yourself that you *don't intend to have sex*! Well, the same is true of
ragged, unsexy, not-ready-for-public-viewing underwear.

Imagine how the ardent lover in the story above must have felt. Here
he had gone to quite a bit of trouble to make this first intimate night
together special and memorable, and his beloved hadn't even cared
enough to wear presentable undies! Granted, she didn't know ahead of
time that he had reserved a room, but she knew they had a date and she
knew in her bones there was a *possibility* that they might become intimate.

Commit this line to memory: **A real Bad Girl *always* wears
underwear that makes her think about sex.** A real Bad Girl wears
lingerie that makes her think about sex *regardless* of whether she actually will or won't be having sex. Perhaps the only thing a Bad Girl and a
Girl Scout have in common is that they share a motto: "Always Be
Prepared." *A Bad Girl doesn't let her underwear close any doors.*

Who's the sexiest guy in the world to you? Is it Tom Cruise? Mel
Gibson? Brad Pitt? Harrison Ford? Your husband? (Lucky you!)
Whoever it is, I want you to keep a picture of him in mind as you com-
plete the first exercise in this chapter.

exercise 1:

The Panty Toss

In this exercise, we are going to mercilessly evaluate your many articles of most personal wear and eliminate the dead weight. So open all of the drawers and cabinets where your unmentionables are lying in wait and get ready to stare down and pare down this personal collection of tired, uninspired, half-sexy, past-sexy, unsexy, and a-sexy stuff.

> Here's the criterion: If you wouldn't want to be seen in the bra, panty, slip, or camisole in question by your personal choice for the sexiest man alive—**Toss it!**

It really is that simple. Why should you ever wear something any less sexy than you would want to wear for a rendezvous with one of the most handsome, sexy, desirable men on the planet? Life is way too short to wear ugly undies! Imagine how sexy you would *always* feel if you kept yourself dressed and groomed to the degree you would want to be dressed and groomed for a tryst with your sexiest man.

I am constantly amazed at how blind we women can become to our underwear. Just for fun sometimes, when I have a class of only women, I'll ask my students to bring in the ugliest pair of underwear they own. I do this for a couple of reasons; the first reason is to wake them up to their ability to go to sleep around this issue. I mean, yikes! If you consider that what they brought in for this exercise is probably their second- or third-ugliest pair because they were too embarrassed to bring in the absolute ugliest . . . "Houston, we have a problem."

I also find it interesting that the most confident, assertive women in my classes invariably come empty-handed; they don't consider any of their underwear ugly.

It's obvious that the scene I used to open this chapter is a Bad Girl "don't." A graduate from the School of Bad wouldn't have those garments in her possession, not to mention on her person. One of the fastest, easiest, most effective ways to feel sexy, sultry, and smokin' hot is by wearing fabulous lingerie. The great thing about your undergarments is that no one knows what you're wearing except you, so you can make the transition from cotton briefs to black lace literally overnight and no one has to be the wiser; unless you want them to!

So if it isn't something you can imagine Mel Gibson peeling off with his teeth, burn it, toss it, or rip it into shreds. But do yourself a really big favor and make it history!

Closet Cleaning, Part 2

Remember the story of Sandy at the beginning of this chapter? Even at the height of her sexual desire, she wasn't aware that she was being sabotaged by her clothing, which was sending a message to her lover that completely neutralized all of the fiery signals she was otherwise communicating.

Instead of the flannel nightie and the bunny slippers, if Sandy showed up in the bedroom in something short, black, and just a bit transparent, do you think she would be sending a clear, *consistent* message to her partner? Do you think she would have a better chance of fulfilling her wish to be ravaged? It's hard to be perceived as Bad when you're dressing like a Girl Scout or like your lover's little sister.

exercise 2:

The Terminator

It's time to get ruthless in the closet. It's time to go through every stitch of clothing you own: the skirts, the blouses, the suits, the casualwear, and the nightgowns.

It's time to try it all on and give it the Bad Girl test: **Does the article of clothing in question *help* or *hinder* your desire to be Bad?** As you consider each item, there are three important questions you have to ask yourself:

- Does this item of clothing make me feel sexy, powerful, in control, and hot?
- Have I worn this item in the past year?
- Is this item of clothing in good repair?

Obviously our goal here is to weed out the clothes that de-sex you in any way. Flannels and bunny slippers like the ones that Sandy wore may be cute, but ask any man and he will tell you that "cute" is not hot. Cute is not dangerous. Cute is not Bad. Cute people are not considered powerful, either. Cute is non-threatening and *young*. It's time to act your age.

Second, if you haven't worn something in over a year, your inner wisdom is clearly trying to tell you something. A year is a long time. If you haven't worn something in 365 days, it's time to let it go. Something better will take its place—I promise!

Third, nothing is less Bad than stained clothes, clothes with frayed cuffs, missing buttons, and broken zippers. A Bad Girl has her act together and makes sure that the clothes she wears reflect the care she takes of herself. If you can't mend it, dump it.

So here's the gauntlet each item of clothing in your closet has to pass:

- If you can answer "yes" to question one (i.e., the article of clothing makes you feel sexy, powerful, and hot)
- And you can answer "yes" to at least one of the other two questions (I've worn the item in the past year or the item is in good repair or can be mended)
- Then you can keep the article of clothing. However, if you can only answer affirmatively to one of the questions, then congratulations! You've just added another item to your "give-away" pile!

As you proceed through this exercise, here's a word of caution for:

- **Closet Cleos:** You want to beware of clothing that falls into the "nice" category. Are you in the dark over what qualifies as a "nice" outfit? Any outfit that your mother would completely approve of. Any outfit that *wouldn't* raise an eyebrow or two at a PTA meeting. Any outfit that doesn't make you think of SEX. Now, don't panic on me, Cleos. Sexy doesn't have to be over-the-top (in fact, it rarely is). You can dress sexy and still be on the understated side. Sexy doesn't have to scream to get noticed. But "nice" isn't hot, "nice" isn't powerful, "nice" isn't sexy. "Nice" is sexless and boring. It's obvious you know how to do nice; we're not worried about that. What you want to explore is the not-so-nice side of you. You know the side of you I'm talking about: the side of you that doesn't smile sunnily, the side of you that doesn't aim to please, the side of you that doesn't do windows! *That's* the direction in which you want to push *your* envelope.

- **Ms. Trees:** You and Closet Cleo are heading for the same destination on this one, you're just coming from opposite directions. What *you* are looking for in an article of clothing is something that makes you *feel* something—and that something is the feeling of being out of uniform, being real, being a woman. You see, I know a secret about the Ms. Trees of the world: Ms. Trees are often extremely shy and vulnerable women. They have been known to use their outlandish clothing and accessories as a shield to hide behind. The sexiest thing a Ms. Tree can do is to shed some of the excess to let people see who you really are. What you are aiming for is a more pared down, simple, less complicated look. *YOU want to get noticed before your clothing gets noticed.* A good rule of thumb for a Ms. Tree is this: If it sparkles, glitters, glows in the dark, or hangs out your body parts like excess produce in an open market, get rid of it! Let the phrase "Less is more" be your guide.

There is a saying from the '60s that goes, "If you're not part of the solution, you're part of the problem." Well, that's the yardstick that needs to be used for any item of clothing hanging in your closet: If it *contributes* to your feeling sexy and being Bad, it's part of the solution. But if it takes away from that feeling (even a little bit, there is no room for half-stepping here), it's part of the problem. Put it up for adoption!

You may wind up with only 50 percent of your clothes remaining. In my opinion, if you have 50 percent of your clothes left, you're doing pretty well. But instead of looking at it as only having half of the clothes you started with, ask yourself:

> *Would I rather keep 50 percent of the clothes I currently have, but feel good 100 percent of the time wearing them? Or, would I rather keep 100 percent of the clothes I currently have but only feel good 50 percent of the time that I wear them?*

The Good Girl's Guide to Bad Girl Sex

A Bad Girl Doesn't Have to Have a Lot of Clothes— Just the Right Ones

Thinking about "the right clothes" vs. "the wrong clothes" reminds me of a great story I'd like to share with you.

One of my best friends is a gorgeous woman and a vice president at a big midwestern bank. I'm in awe of everything about her . . . except the way she dresses! It's not that she has bad taste, she's just terribly formal most of the time. There's nothing wrong with pinstripes and worsted woolens on a banker during the day, but on a date? So when she came out to California to visit me once, I was secretly thrilled when the airline lost her luggage. I tried to convince her that it was a case of divine intervention and that she should embrace the opportunity to buy some new clothes. But being a banker (read: frugal), she was content to borrow jeans and T-shirts from me. She got away with that until we bumped into a neighbor of mine who invited us to a party he was throwing for himself at his country club, to celebrate his promotion to partner in his firm. So much for blue jeans and T-shirts!

Jody decided that she would just wear something of mine—figuring that if she was going to be uncomfortable in something, she didn't want the added insult of having to pay for it. So the evening of the big shindig rolls around and Jody pretty much just covers her eyes and grabs something out of my closet sight unseen.

And what a fortuitous grab it turned out to be! The "something" my friend landed on turned out to be a sultry little red number that I hadn't even worn yet (harrumph!) It was sleeveless on one side, with a deep décolletage which accented her breasts in the most stunning way (breasts I didn't even know she had!). The silky fabric hugged her curves like a Porsche on the Swiss Alps, the color was great on her, and I knew right then and there I'd better say good-bye to that outfit because I was never going to get it back! She looked like another person. I had never seen her so sexy and self-assured. What was especially amazing to me is that I could tell that she could feel it.

We went to the party and my uptight friend Jody was the belle of the ball. I had never seen her so flirtatious and relaxed. Having to reach outside of her usual wardrobe choices forced her to try something new. It forced her to go in a direction that, under usual circumstances, she never would have considered. I also think that it helped that she was among people who didn't know her; people who had no preconceived notions of her; people who didn't know she usually had a stick up her butt! She got to try on a new persona free of charge, to speak. She felt free to try something new because if she fell flat on her face, she would never have to see any of those people again. Still, I know it was the dress that made the big difference.

Before Jody left, she paid me the ultimate compliment by asking me to take her to a few of my favorite boutiques and help her find some clothes of her own. I'm sure she'll still be in pinstripes from nine to five, but maybe now, that extra button on her blouse will be left undone. It does my heart good to know that, at least after hours, she'll be exploring that relaxed, sensual, vibrant side of herself a lot more often.

Ring in the New!

By now I'm assuming you've weeded out all of the undesirables from your closet. This really is a very important step and I hope you won't shortchange yourself by not doing it. By cleaning out your closet, not only are you physically making room for new clothes, but you are also doing a mental clearing away of the associations you have to who you were when you wore those clothes. You are making room "psychically" for a paradigm shift to take place within you. It's time to open the windows, both literally and figuratively, and let the excitement of possibility air out your closet and your mind.

Now *What Do You Wear?*

When you finish these closet-cleaning exercises you're left with clothes that make you feel good, but there's a lot of empty space on the rod. What are you going to fill it with? What direction should you go in now?

Even if money isn't a consideration for you, I suggest you start your wardrobe replacement slowly. Just as you wouldn't enter the Indianapolis 500 the same week you get your driver's license, you would be putting unrealistic expectations on yourself to try to go from where you are now to 100 percent "Frederick's of Hollywood" in one afternoon.

In the following exercise, you're going to use the powers of imagination and creative visualization to help determine what *your* Bad Girl would wear if she were given free rein. Where you're going there are no "shoulda's," "woulda's," or "coulda's." There is no one to answer to, and no one to embarrass.

Keeping the story of my friend Jody in mind as your inspiration, I'm going to ask you to let yourself wander. It's time to dream a little dream. Great athletes practice their moves over and over again in their minds before going out on the court or on the slopes. They *visualize* the desired result in order to make it happen.

You're going to use the same technique the athletes use to help you shape your new wardrobe. Before you actually buy a stitch of clothes, you are first going to *see* yourself in a whole new way. Using creative visualization, you're going on a virtual shopping spree—and your Bad side gets to pick out the clothes!

exercise 3:

Virtually Shop Till You Drop

- Sit or lie in a comfortable position. Turn off your cell phone, your pager, or any other device that might intrude on your private time.

- Breathe deeply through your nose and into your belly. Let your stomach rise slowly with the air. Breathe out through your mouth. Take as many breaths as you need to feel deeply relaxed.

- Now imagine that you're in a place where no one knows you. Maybe, like my friend Jody, you're at a party with a group of people you've never met before. Maybe you've moved to a new town in order to make a fresh start. Maybe you're on vacation in a city you've never been to before; or a foreign country! Or maybe you got lucky and the airline lost your luggage and is giving you money to replace all your clothes. Whatever it is, make it real for yourself. Just remember that in your visualization there are no consequences, so you are free to really play fast and loose. No one is judging you, comparing you, shaming, or pigeonholing you. The only rule for this exercise is that whatever you wear has to make you feel like a hottie! With the brakes off, the regulators bypassed, and the censors bound and gagged: **How would you dress?**

- Here's your chance to try on that skintight purple leather dress you eyeballed on the mannequin in the storefront window. Maybe you've always loved the Italian designers, so in your visualization you've moved to Rome. You develop a penchant for high heels and hip-hugging skirts that start above the knee. You pair them with a tight, white blouse which you wear with the collar up and unbuttoned just enough for the top edge of your lacy bra to show. **See yourself** walking down the street in the outfit. **See yourself** at work. **See yourself** having dinner. You move with a feline's grace; you wear your clothes with pleasure and style.

- Maybe you're a sun worshipper so in your fantasy you're in Florida or California. Your light tan looks spectacular with vivid oranges, violets, and greens. Your daily walks have really toned up your tummy and you've taken to wearing halter tops and low slung jeans that show off your belly button. **See** yourself strolling along the oceanfront completely relaxed in your sexy attire. **Feel** the confidence and pleasure with which you move. **Watch** the gentle rolling of your hips as you saunter down the boulevard.

- Or you're at a nightclub in the south of France. You're wearing black polyurethane pants that look as if they were painted onto your body. You've fashioned a top out of an expensive silk scarf that you've wrapped around your torso and tied behind your neck. You also have on big gold hoop earrings. Your hair is free and loose. You're on a crowded dance floor having the time of your life. You feel the music deep inside you and you let it express itself through your body.

But all of these are *my* fantasies. What are yours? Let your visualizations rise to the surface of your mind like bubbles in champagne. You're not committing yourself to dressing in all of the various ways you appear, so really pry those fantasies loose; you're getting acquainted with a part of yourself that has been in deep cover for a very long time. As you see yourself in the various locales, doing a variety of activities, look closely at yourself:

- **What kind shoes are you wearing?** Shoes are as important as the clothing itself. You can feel like a "ten" from the ankles up, but with the wrong footwear, it can drag the whole ensemble down. Make sure your shoes make you feel as fabulous as your clothes do.

- **What does your hair look like?** Is it longer than it currently is? Is it shorter? Is it a different color? Hair is one of the easiest things a woman can change about herself; *and* one of the most dramatic. Pay close attention to the way your hair appears in your visualizations.

- **How does your makeup look?** Are you wearing a shade of lipstick that's unusual for you? Is it unusual for you to be wearing lipstick at all? Are your eyebrows artfully arched and darkened? Are you wearing less makeup, more makeup, no makeup? What direction does your Bad Girl want to go in?

After you have virtually shopped till you've dropped and you've explored every road not taken from a fashion point of view, take some time to review and reflect. If you're keeping a Bad Girl journal, jot down:

- **What kind of clothes did you wear during this visualization?** How did they differ from what you wear now? *Be specific.* Were they tighter, shorter, more dressy, more casual? Did they feature any part of your anatomy more prominently?

- **When you visualized yourself wearing the clothes:** Did you move differently? Hold yourself differently? Were you smiling? Smoldering? Did you look self-conscious? Were you able to relax into it?

- **And finally, ask yourself:** What is stopping me from dressing this way *now?* What's holding me back?

Make a list of all the reasons why you "can't" dress the way you saw yourself in your visualizations. Are there practical reasons? For example, if you live in Alaska, you're probably not going to get the opportunity to wear tube tops that often. But temperature considerations aside, what are the reasons that present themselves and convince you that you "can't" dress in a sexy, powerful, age-appropriate manner?

Don't try telling me (or yourself) that it's the same ten or twenty pounds you keep trying to lose that's stopping you. If you need examples, look at the actress Camryn Manheim, or the plus-sized model Emme. Both are very full-figured women who know that life isn't a dress rehearsal; they aren't *waiting* until they hit a certain weight before they allow themselves to feel sexy and good about themselves. They are big, Bad, and beautiful *right now!*

You say you don't have the money? Even most mid-sized cities today have consignment shops where the rich and/or famous place their once- or twice-worn garments in order to sell them at deeply discounted prices. Also, most major department stores offer discounts upon discounts at the end of each season. You'll be buying summer clothing at the beginning of the fall season (or vice versa), but as long as it's an item that makes you feel sizzling hot, it will always be in season.

My suspicion is that most of you will cite the fear of disapproval from someone in your life—either significant or insignificant—who you *believe* will have a problem with you if your style of dress changes. Now, if you're worried about the other soccer moms, I have four little words for you that will set you free: *they'll get over it!* Sure, you may be the subject of some petty gossip for a week or two, but trust me when I tell you that they are far more concerned with themselves and their own problems than the fact that you've taken to wearing push-up bras and French T-shirts. They'll soon forget you ever dressed any other way!

On the other hand, if you are in a committed relationship and you're worried about how the man in your life might react to the change in you, that obviously will require more serious attention.

I heartily support the notion of talking with him beforehand and letting him know your motivation for the changes you're contemplating making. You may want to show him this book; let him look it over and encourage him to ask you questions. Let him know that you are doing this work for yourself (and not to attract someone new). Reassure him that it is your intention to bring the new discoveries, the new excitement, and the new heat, right back into your relationship with him. If you find he is still skeptical, ask him to give you a 90 day "try out" period. Ask him to hold his tongue, his opinions, and his judgments for at least 90 days while you follow the program in this book. If after that time he still has questions or concerns, you will agree to sit down with him to talk them over. But if he's in seventh heaven with the new woman in his life, the deadline will come and go without anybody even noting its passing.

I hope I've touched on the top three objections you may have come up with as to why you "can't" dress more like a Bad Girl. Remind yourself that you can and should go slowly. It would be a shock to your system to start dressing in a completely different manner overnight. That's why you start building your new wardrobe with *your own clothes*—the clothes you already own that support your experience of yourself as a powerfully sexual person. You can then use your visualizations as a jumping-off point from which to start adding new clothes.

Mystery Shopper

It's time to transform the virtual shopping spree you went on earlier into a real shopping spree. But before you start hyperventilating, two things:

> **Thing #1:** You don't have to spend any money if you don't want to (but I bet you will!).

Bad Girls Dress the Part

Thing #2: You're **not allowed** to shop at a store, dress shop, or boutique where you would usually go. You *must* go to an unfamiliar store. You get to be a Mystery Shopper.

If you're a Closet Cleo and you usually shop at Talbot's, Banana Republic, or the Gap, I want you to pick a store that usually makes you ask yourself, "Who the heck shops at this place?" It may be a "Victoria's Secret" type store (or catalogue), or a local store in your neighborhood mall that carries more risqué outerwear.

If you're a Ms. Christmas Tree who usually does her shopping at all of the places Closet Cleo avoids like the plague, I want you to find a store that heretofore held absolutely no interest for you. It could be one of those that you usually pass by and say to yourself, "Borrrringggg!" It might even be a classic Cleo store! You want to be looking for clothes that can be worn to give the *suggestion* of sex, not clothes that tell the entire story.

What I am trying to recreate for you is the experience my friend Jody had when she reached blindly into my closet and came out with a completely new look for herself. I want you to go to a store where virtually everything hanging on the racks is going to be different from anything you have at home.

Part of being a Mystery Shopper is going to a store where no one will know you. Remember how Jody didn't know anyone (except for me) at the party? By remaining anonymous, you get to experiment with this new side of yourself without worrying what your regular salesperson might say, or running into someone you know when you step out of the dressing room. Go across town; go to *another* town if you want to. Do whatever you need to do to be comfortable during this process.

And by all means pick a store (or catalogue) that supports the style of clothing you wore in your virtual shopping spree. The time has come to convert that "out of body" experience into an "in body" experience. It's time to try your Bad Girl on for size.

exercise 4:

Actual Shopping Spree

- With your list of clothing that your Bad Girl chose during your earlier visualizations in hand, head out for the appropriate store for you, as described above, depending on your type (Cleo or Tree).

- If you feel brave enough, find a friendly salesperson and tell her that you are interested in trying on some new looks. If you're a Ms. Tree, let her know that you're trying to simplify your look, but you want it to be very sexy, clean, and lean. And if you're a Cleo, let her know that you tend to dress conservatively, and you want to try on things that are edgier, more dangerous, and very, very sexy.

- If you're not ready for human interaction, that's okay, too. Using the same criteria I've outlined above, pick out some clothes on your own and head for the dressing room.

You've cleaned out your closet and made room for it in both your closet and in your head. You've tried it on in the privacy of your own mind. And now, finally, you're actually wearing it: your unique, 100 percent yours, Bad Girl outfit. How does it feel? How do you look? Are you loving it? Will it take some getting used to? Or are you taking to it like a duck to water?

- If you don't like the first thing you try on, keep going until you find something you do like. It's a big store; you'll find *something*.

- But if you're having difficulty relaxing into one of the new looks, pretend you're a model who has been paid a lot of money to make the clothing look its best. Don't comment on it; don't editorialize. If you're giggling, stop. Make an entrance. Sell the look. Take it seriously. Now how do you feel? Did that bit of role playing help you lose your self-consciousness? Were you able to step outside of yourself for a moment or two and see yourself as a stranger might?

- If you haven't done so already, it's time to talk to a salesperson. If you love the way you look, you deserve some validation. If you have qualms, you deserve a second opinion!

Shopping Spree Wrap-Up

I hope you've found at least one item you've fallen completely in love with. If for some reason you haven't found anything you adore, try another store. It could be you're just not in the right place. If you go to a second store and you still can't find anything that fits the bill, it could be you need to revise your criteria a bit. Maybe you're trying to push too far too fast. If so, bump it down a notch or two. Dressing Bad is supposed to be fun! If it ever starts to feel scary or threatening, you're probably going way beyond your comfort and safety zone. If so, dress it down a little bit until you're back in a place that you can handle.

Becoming Visible

Now that you've found a great new piece or two (or three, or four!), prepare to share it with the world! That's right, you've had plenty of time hiding your light beneath a bushel; it's time to let it shine!

Within *one week* of buying your new clothes, I want you to wear either one of the items (if you bought separates), or one of the outfits in *public*. If it's appropriate for your work, wear it to work. If it's more of an after-hours garment, wear it out to dinner, to a party, or on a date.

I consider myself pretty fortunate in the wardrobe department because no one in their right mind would ever tell me that I'm dressed inappropriately for the office! Being a sex therapist gives you a lot of room—you need to be professional, of course, but you don't need to be buttoned up like a business school student. But *you* may not have the same type of freedom where you work. Please take your particular situation into consideration when dressing for your job. A little bit of common sense can go a long way. Every situation is unique and only you know where the line dividing pushing the envelope and going over the top lies. I would hate for you to make a misstep or put your job in jeopardy by dressing inappropriately for work.

If the Shoe Fits . . .

Have you ever heard the saying that you can tell how well-off a person is by looking at her shoes? In these modern times we don't have the same barometers of wealth that were common a century ago; men and women don't wear hats every time they step out of doors, and women don't wear gloves and veils. To a large extent, especially when dressing casually, we all look pretty much the same.

Except when it comes to shoes. A well-dressed woman would never wear cheap or worn out shoes. *Nothing*, absolutely *nothing*, detracts from the over-all look of an outfit more than marred, dull, or tattered footwear.

exercise 5:
Take an Inventory of Your Shoes

It's time to show the same ruthlessness toward your shoes that you managed to show toward your wardrobe and your lingerie.

That "great deal" you bought on sale, but are too tight? Pitch 'em! Those espadrilles you bought in Spain that are slowly disintegrating? Toss 'em! The favorite pair of pumps with the broken strap? Replace 'em! Use the one-year rule again as your guide: If you haven't worn the shoes during the previous 365 days, out they go.

Just so you don't think I'm completely without a heart, I do believe that some shoes can be successfully rehabilitated. Maybe they just need new soles or heels; or a professional polishing. But I think you will find that your more expensive shoes respond the best to regular upkeep. It's been my experience that the cheaper the shoe, the shorter the life. Spend a little more on your shoes and keep them in good repair; you will find that you get a much better return on your investment. Besides, you're just plain worth it!

The Cherry on Top

In this last segment of this chapter, we're going to talk about the icing on the cake (and the cherry on top): makeup and hair. Makeup and hair are tricky. They can be our greatest assets or our greatest enemies. They can accentuate our best features, or bring attention to our worst flaws. Our hair and makeup can date us or make us timeless.

I've known women who will buy new clothing every year without fail, but they haven't changed their hair or makeup during the past decade. Are you one of these women? When was the last time you made a significant change in either category?

Second, how *flexible* is your "look"? By flexible, I mean do you have a sense of fun with your hair and makeup? Do you use them like the accessories they are? Or do you just wear your hair one way and your makeup one way all the time? All day, every day, day in, day out; day after day after day . . . ho hum. You get my drift.

Third, how W-O-M-A-N is your look? Are you still playing the girl next door with your hair piled up on your head so cute, cute, cute, like you just came back from the laundromat? Are you always going for that wholesome or careful look? I'll say it once again: Cute is not Bad. Wholesome is not Bad. Nice is not Bad. And careful is not Bad. These looks aren't going to start any fires.

It's time to shake and wake! Shake things up and wake up the senses! If you've never treated yourself (or been treated) to a makeover, *that's* about to change! I'm talking about one of those all-day, "I usually only give these as gifts" kind of makeovers.

Most spas and salons have a full day package of services that they offer at a reduced price. This is a good thing, because you want "the works!" Now is the perfect time to rethink your whole look; to get a hot new haircut and learn a few new ways to apply makeup.

We all know how a "bad hair day" can ruin our outlook and erode our self-confidence. Turning that truism on its head, it should also be true that a great hair and makeup day should brighten our outlook and boost our self-confidence. Of course, this is absolutely true. A Bad Girl understands the important role that feeling good and looking good play in being Bad. She knows the difference between a bad hair day and a *Bad* hair day (*Bad* being sexy, hot, edgy, new). *Being* Bad is all about feeling *good*. Really good. "Like a million bucks" good. From head to toe good.

So, no excuses. *Just do it.* You will love yourself for it. The more you love yourself, the better you feel. And the better you feel, the Badder you get!

Chapter 4

Bad Girls Walk the Walk

I see it all the time and frankly, it makes me a little nuts: A beautiful woman who has the potential to be so hot, but her presentation says, "Don't look at me; I'm a dud." She can be wearing something that's saying exactly the opposite—a skirt that's slit to the thigh, a halter that shows off her beautiful breasts, or a thong that turns every head on the beach—but when you look at her closely, you lose all interest. It may be her posture or the way that she walks. It may be the expression on her face or the fact that she's cracking her gum. It could be all of these things, or none of these things. But *something* she's doing just *isn't working* and she leaves a trail of disinterest in her wake.

Take a walk around your favorite city on any given day and you'll see exactly what I mean. So many women *trying* to look alluring, yet it looks like one boring parts display because the owners of these parts seem so disconnected from their sexual power. What is it that's missing? It's not the equipment. What's missing is the ability to feel *connected* to that equipment, and the ability to offer it seductively for other people's pleasure (not to mention her own). Without that connection, the allure is lost. Breasts are just breasts. Thighs are just thighs. Curves become uninteresting, and the jumble of parts is all quickly forgettable. It's an "out of body" experience that way too many women suffer from, and, to be completely blunt, it turns men off.

Then there will be one woman who immediately stands out—the woman who is noticed and who everyone remembers. She may not be any prettier, any more fit, or any more buxom than anyone else in the room. Her clothes may not be any more expensive or stylish. And yet, she has a way of carrying herself that makes men pay attention. Her sexual power is palpable. This is the woman that you can be, and it doesn't take a miracle to get you there.

In the previous chapter we talked about the clothes you need to make the woman. In this chapter, we're going to talk about the *woman* you need to make the woman, with a focus on what I call **sexual alignment.** The way you walk, the way you sit, the way you enter and exit a room. The way you hold your shoulders, the way you move your arms; where you rest your hands and how you cross your legs. Your pace, your posture, your focus; *everything* has an impact.

What do people see when they watch you approaching? What is the picture you present to the world and how can you make that image one that won't be forgotten? We're talking packaging here, we're talking gestalt—the larger picture that makes a man want you. If you want to be Bad, you have to *live* the part, and let it show in every gesture. *That* is what it means to walk the walk.

Shimmy Shimmy Coco Pop!

Truman Capote is one of my favorite authors. He and Marilyn Monroe were friends, and in an article he once wrote, he spoke of an uncanny experience he once had with Marilyn.

In the article, he speaks of going to a funeral with Marilyn. She was very upset by the death of her friend and cried into her handkerchief throughout the eulogy. After the service, on the sidewalk outside of the New York City funeral home, she took Capote's arm and they began to walk. No one, not one soul, looked at them as they walked slowly arm in arm. Suddenly, as if revived by the air, Marilyn asked Capote, "Want to see something funny?" Capote couldn't imagine what she was referring to, but answered, "Of course." (I mean, who wouldn't?) Suddenly, Marilyn squared her shoulders, lifted her chin, tightened her belly, shortened her step, and *immediately*, within seconds, passersby were gawking, staring, nudging, pointing, and waving. "Look, look, it's Marilyn!," they said.

Capote was stunned. Same woman, same clothes, same tear-streaked face. She hadn't even removed her sunglasses or the scarf from her head. But it wasn't just the change in her posture or her gait; Capote saw a radiance emanating from her that a moment earlier was nowhere to be seen—we might refer to it today as someone's aura. He saw that the actress had the ability to turn "Marilyn" on and off at will. She could disappear inside herself when necessary and reappear when it pleased her to do so. "That's the power of Marilyn," the legend is reported having said. What can you say, except, amen to that.

So how in the world did she do it? How did she tap into that power? Don't misunderstand me—I'm not suggesting that we can all be Marilyn Monroes, or that we even should be; but I am suggesting that we can all study Marilyn Monroe and learn from her. Whether you are a fan of Marilyn Monroe or not, there is no arguing that her sex appeal has proved to be enduring beyond all imagination. She was a woman who could "walk the walk" with the best of them.

Who's That Girl?

Important Question #1:
How do you walk through the world?

Do you walk in such a way that when you enter a room men ask their friends, "Who's that girl?" Or is it more likely to be, "What girl?" after you've made your exit. Do people often tell you to slow down? To hurry up? Has anyone ever said to you, "I knew that was you coming," when they heard your step before seeing you? Did you ask them how they knew, or were you too scared to learn the answer?

Important Question #2:
Where is your focus when you walk?

Do you stay completely in your head and try not to think about the fact that you're walking at all? Do you focus on your feet? Are you focusing on your arms wrapped around your purse because you're afraid someone will steal it?

I'll let you in on a little known secret: other people in your environment (this includes men) will focus on whatever it is you are focusing on about yourself. This fact is a two-edged sword, but it can be a wonderful thing, *if* you know how to use it to your benefit. That's what this chapter is all about: learning how to use some basic body language techniques so that they're all working *for* you, instead of against you.

Smile, You're on Candid Camera!

There is only one way for you to see how you look when you walk, talk, and enter a room, and that is by having someone videotape you. Hey! Where do you think you're going?! Don't get cold feet now, the *real* fun's just beginning! Okay, the truth is that I know a certain percentage of you will just skim over the next few pages and never actually do this exercise, but for those of you who take this next exercise seriously, I cannot tell you how richly rewarded you will be. You will glean insights into your personal presentation that might otherwise have remained hidden from you forever.

Consider this: Do you know someone who is always getting derailed after the third or fourth date? Maybe that "someone" is you. If you have been hitting the same baffling roadblocks over and over again in the early stages of a relationship, it may be because you are sending nonverbal communications that are at cross purposes with your stated goal of getting closer with the object of your desire. This exercise may just be the key to solving the mystery for you.

Or maybe this is a more familiar scenario: You spend hours getting dressed for an evening out, carefully applying your makeup and getting your hair "just-so." Your date picks you up, or you arrive at the party, and what's the first thing you hear? "You look *cute!*" *Cute.* Ugh. Whoever is delivering the "compliment" means only the best by it, but here you are, hoping you look hot, hoping you look devastating, and all you get is "cute."

Walking like a Bad Girl will shut down the "cutes" forever. It can be done. You can learn it, but first, you have to *earn* it. You have to be brave enough to face the truth of the situation as it exists right now. So go grab a video camera and a trusted friend, and start walking!

exercise 1:

Strutting Your Stuff

The person behind the camera is an important factor in this exercise. The best scenario would be to have a friend who is also reading this book and who is also currently enrolled in the Bad Girl training program. Short of that, a good friend who supports your desire to grow and change (be it a girl friend, a platonic boyfriend, or your husband or lover) is the person you want to tap for this exercise.

Explain ahead of time that you don't need a director, and you're not looking for a coach. At this stage all you need is a human camera holder, although you may be asking for more input from them later. But right now, you just want to capture yourself on videotape walking, sitting, and standing as naturally as possible. Please keep the following points in mind:

- You're going to walk at two speeds for this exercise. First, you'll walk at a leisurely pace while your camera operator tapes you. Very simple. Depending on the time of year, you may want to conduct this exercise at an indoor mall (the store windows will provide a good distraction for you and will keep you from becoming too self-conscious). Or, if the weather permits, you can go to a local park.

- Your camera operator should be far enough away to allow you to walk towards him or her for at least forty feet or so before you pass.

- *Forget the camera is there.* Try to think of *anything* but the camera and how you are walking. Get lost in thought. Try not to look at the camera; look in a few store windows if you're at the mall, or at the scenery if you're outdoors.

- After you've walked for a few minutes, take a seat. Cross and uncross your legs a few times. Keep the tape running.

- Now stand up. Have your camera operator *video-tape you from behind,* walking away from him/her.

- Now turn around and walk *briskly* back toward the camera. This time, walk as though your parking meter is about to expire. Don't stroll; walk with a firm purpose.

- Make sure your camera operator videotapes you from behind walking at this pace, too.

Reviewing the Tape

The First Viewing: Watch the tape you have just made at the speed it was recorded. Next, consider the following questions:

- **What is your over-all impression of your walk?**
  Do you look coordinated? Wobbly? Approachable? Off-putting? Do *you* like the way you walk? If you don't like the way you walk, it's a pretty sure bet that you aren't turning on anyone else, either.

- **What part of your body do you *lead* with?**
  To determine the part of the body that you lead with, look for the part of you that looks as though some-one might be pulling on a string that is attached to that point. For example, if you lead with your head, you're looking down, to some degree. If you lead with your shoulders, you're going to look hunched over. If you lead with your knees, you probably look as if you're leaning backward a bit. If you lead with your stomach, your pelvis is tilted forward and you may doing a bit of a duckwalk.
  If you can't name a body part that you lead with, what you do may be extremely subtle; you may not be able to pick up on anything right away. Or you may be one of the lucky few who has a neutral walk. Person-ally, I've always had a tendency to lead with my chest. A chest-walker's body language gives the impression that she is assertive and possibly aggressive; we'll talk

more about body language later. For now, run your assessment of your walk by your camera buddy to see if he or she agrees with that assessment.

• **What are your arms doing?**
Are they stiff at your sides? Does one swing and one stay stationary? Are you clutching them across your chest? Arms are a vitally important and often over-looked element in the way we walk. What's going on with *your* arms?

• **How do you look "going"?**
You've had a chance to evaluate how you look com-ing, but how do you look going? What does the back of your head look like? Is your hair in place? Is your sweater pulled down evenly? Do your elbows make "chicken wings" from behind? These may seem like silly questions, but a bad presentation from the rear has the same affect as dragging toilet paper on your shoe: Everyone notices it, but no one has the guts to tell you. Make checking your rear view in the mirror a daily part of your dressing ritual.

• **What happens when you walk fast?**
I'm willing to bet money that walking fast feels a whole lot more natural to a large number of you. It's especially likely if you originally categorized your-self as a Cleo. Although you would think it would be the opposite, rushing actually makes you *less* visi-ble. Women who are uncomfortable being seen, who are disconnected from their sexual core, and who are literally out of step with their own sensual speed and rhythm, rush. We all have a legitimate reason to get a move on from time to time, but a Bad Girl does not make a habit of it. What else do you notice about yourself at this speed? Does your walk change when you're rushing? Do you hunker down like a linebacker going for the touchdown? If so, isn't that reason enough to stop?

- **Do any repetitive gestures or tics jump out at you?**
  Are you constantly smoothing your hair behind one ear, biting your bottom lip, picking at your cuticles, or doing any other funny or strange things with your nose, mouth, hair, eyes, etc.? At normal playback, you may not even notice anything. Our tics are usually so ingrained, we often have trouble even seeing them. If nothing pops out at you right away, that's okay—don't force it. You may be relatively "tic-free" or, you may see something later during the all-important second viewing.

The Second Viewing: I know that this might sound a bit odd. But this time I want you to watch your tape on fast-forward with the audio turned down. If you need to, watch it this way more than once. Now consider these questions:

- **If you had difficulty telling before, can you now see what part of your body you lead with?**
  Speeding up the tape makes a lot of information more clear, doesn't it?

- **What repetitive moves or gestures do you see now?**
  Is anything new popping out at you that you didn't see before? Or is what you saw before simply much more obvious? Can you imagine how many times you make those same gestures in an hour, in a day, *on a date?*

- **What is the effect of the gesture(s)?**
  This is *so* important. Is the gesture distracting? Childish? Annoying? All of the above? Let me elaborate.

  Distracting:
  Constantly touching your face or your hair; frequent scratching of your arm, or your neck. Picking or plucking at yourself. Frequent hair-tossing.

  Annoying:
  Chewing and cracking gum, walking with your arm on your hip, or dragging your feet.

Childish:

Something that little kids do when they are unaware of being watched. Here's a particularly popular one: twisting your hair around your index finger. I feel as though I see this at least once or twice in every class I teach. It's the first class of the semester and one of my new students has obviously put a lot of thought and effort into her outfit; in fact, she is dressed to the nines. But all of a sudden, she grabs a hank of hair with the crook of her index finger and starts twisting it around and around. *Bzzzz!* Thanks for playing! You have just been disqualified as a grown-up. A habit like this is an instant indication that the woman in question isn't *in* her womanhood at all. At that moment, at least, she's still in her little girl.

The strange thing is, under the correct circumstances, any one of these little tics or gestures can actually be sexy and flirtatious. It's when they become unconscious and ritualistic that they lose any allure they may otherwise have. Touching yourself when you're talking to a man can be a very sexy thing to do (even twirling your hair!). **The keys are moderation and *conscious* application of the gesture.** Just as a little perfume is intoxicating, and a lot of perfume is nauseating, the same can be said for self-touch; a little is erotic, too much just looks neurotic! Keep his focus where it belongs—on you!

Is Your Walk Talking Behind Your Back?

Every walk sends a message. I mentioned earlier that left to my own devices, I tend to walk with my chest leading the way, which can make me seem more aggressive and less feminine than I like to be considered. What message does *your* walk convey? Let's take a look at some of the different ways of walking and how your walk may be sending unspoken messages to men in your life.

Leading with your head: If you walk with your head, you're looking down. And when you're looking down, it's very difficult to make eye contact. If you can't make eye contact, you can't connect with anyone. And if you can't connect with anyone, you can't be Bad. Women who are always looking at their feet as they walk are silently saying, "Don't approach me, don't look at me, and whatever you do, don't touch me!" Looking down is the recluse's walk, or the hermit's walk. Whether you mean to or not, when you walk in this manner, you are isolating yourself from those around you, and you are telegraphing a message that tells people to keep their distance. You probably walk at a relatively fast pace too, driving that message home.

Leading with your knees: At its most extreme, walkers who lead with their knees look as though they're on a slant board. When your head is the last part of your anatomy to enter a room, you give the impression of being lackadaisical, reluctant, and apathetic. I'm assuming that isn't the impression you want to convey under any condition. If you're a knees-first kind of woman, you probably walk more slowly than most people. Too slowly. Half-asleep slowly.

Leading with the shoulders: When you lead with your shoulders, you walk around in a kind of turtle's shell. You give the impression that you are shy and fearful. Although (or perhaps because) it looks as though you're trying to protect yourself, you probably attract people who do their best to take advantage of you or dominate you. People who walk this way do so at various speeds.

Leading with the stomach: Besides bearing an uncomfortably close resemblance to Daisy Duck, this walk also comes with a couple of accompanying affectations: You are more likely to shuffle your feet and I'll bet your left or right hand can usually be found dangling from the wrist by your side. This is how toddlers walk when they're first learning to stay upright. It is a very babyish walk. It's a walk that tells people that you are not to be taken seriously; that you are harmless—a pushover (almost literally a pushover, as your center of balance is completely off-kilter when you walk this way). Women who lead with their stomachs can be both fast and slow walkers.

Bad Girls Walk the Walk

Leading with the chest: As I shared with you before, this is the walk I can lapse into when I'm not connecting to my Bad Girl self. It's a kind of macho swagger that I find unappealing in *men*, so you can imagine how I feel about it in women (myself included, of course!). It's not a walk that invites anyone, man or woman, to approach, as it gives the impression that you're a combative person, possibly with a large chip on your shoulder. Walkers who lead with their chests usually aren't in a rush, but no one is rushing to greet you either because you don't make a lot of friends with this walk.

So there you have several of the most common styles of walking, their accompanying speeds, and the subliminal messages they can communicate. Your walk may fall into one of these categories to a greater or lesser degree, or you may combine a few elements from a couple of different walks for something completely unique! Unfortunately, none of these walks qualifies as the good kind of Bad. Fortunately, with a little time, effort, and practice, you *can* change the way you walk. Are you ready to kiss your old, lackluster walk good-bye? Are you ready to have the Baddest walk on the block? Then keep turning those pages.

By George, I Think She's Got It!

Most women will remember that in *My Fair Lady,* Professor Henry Higgins made poor Eliza Doolittle walk around with a stack of books on her head to teach her proper posture and carriage. I've got a faster, easier, and more effective way to correct your posture, focus your energy and attention, and get you walking like a real Bad Girl.

Remember the technique you used to identify which body part you lead with when you walk? You looked for the part of your body that looked as if it was being pulled forward by a string. Do you know which body part a Bad Girl leads with? I'll give you three guesses. Lower . . . lower . . . you've got it! It's the pelvis!

When a Bad Girl walks, she leads with her pelvis. It makes sense, doesn't it? I mean, where else should a Bad Girl's attention be?

Now you know *what* to lead with, but *how* is it done? Unless you're a belly dancer, chances are you're not in the habit of isolating and exercising the pelvic muscles. A limber, well-toned pelvis is an essential element of the Bad Girl's walk; it can also come in handy during a few other activities. Hint. Hint. Hint. But first things first.

If you're like most women over the age of eighteen, your pelvis may very well be frozen in one long solid block with your lower back. This may come as a surprise to you, but your pelvis was meant to have a life of its very own. Your pelvis is connected to your spine through tendons and muscle, not bone, and therefore, those muscles can be stretched and strengthened. A stretched, strengthened pelvis is a beautiful thing!

Here are a couple of simple, yet effective exercises you can do daily to help isolate, strengthen, and tone your pelvis.

exercise 2:

Rockin' . . .

1. Place a towel or mat on the floor. Lie flat on your back. Inhale deeply through your nose. Feel your belly rise with the breath. Let your muscles relax. Exhale through your mouth. Repeat several times.

2. Place your arms, palms down, parallel to your sides.

3. Slide your feet toward your body until your legs form an upside-down "V."

4. Inhale one more time. On the exhale, use your stomach, thigh, and butt muscles to gently **tilt your pelvis and raise it off the floor.** This will raise your bottom off the floor a few inches, but your lower back should stay pressed against the floor.

5. Slowly lower your pelvis back to the floor.

6. Repeat this pelvic rock ten times.

exercise 3:

Risin' . . .

1. Relax on the floor with your legs in a "V" as you did in the first part of this exercise.

2. Tighten your stomach muscles. Take a deep breath. On the exhale, use your thigh muscles and butt muscles to slowly **raise your pelvis and your lower back off the floor.** Imagine a string pulling your pelvis up toward the ceiling.

3. Hold for two counts, then lower your pelvis back to the floor.

4. Repeat the lifts for a set of ten. On the tenth lift, **raise and hold for a count of five.** Then slowly lower your pelvis to the floor. Rest. Do a second set.

Rolling Thunder

The next exercise requires an inflatable exercise ball. These balls are really gaining in popularity. They're inexpensive, effective, and it's like having a complete gym in the privacy of your own home. You can find the balls at your local sports equipment store, at a "Relax the Back" store, or on the Internet. I entered the term *exercise balls* on my favorite search engine and came up with several sites that sell the balls. One site called "Just Balls," had excellent prices and a wide selection. The balls come in different sizes for different heights, so be sure to order the correct size.

Also, unless you get lucky and you find one that's already inflated, you will need a small pump to blow the thing up. Once again, I found an inexpensive hand pump for sale on the Internet site I mentioned above. Once it's inflated, you should be able to sit on your ball without feeling as though you're sinking deeply into it, but it shouldn't be so tight that it feels as if it's about to explode, either. Somewhere between those two extremes is the firmness you are aiming for.

exercise 4:

. . . and Rollin'

1. Sit up straight on your ball, with your feet planted firmly in front of you, about a foot apart.

2. Rest your hands on your knees.

3. Tighten your abdominal muscles and slowly tuck and roll your pelvis forward. Your feet and legs should stay still. Your shoulders and torso should also remain fairly still. It isn't necessary to make this a large movement; a small tuck and roll is sufficient to get the maximum benefit. Hold for one count.

4. Roll your pelvis back to the center.

5. Now, roll your pelvis back. Be careful not to collapse the abdominal muscles with this move; the temptation is to let those muscles go, but keep them tight as you roll a few inches toward the rear.

6. Come back to center. Roll forward and backward in this manner ten times.

Now switch to a side-to-side motion.

1. Sitting up straight and holding your stomach tight, rest your hands on your knees and roll the ball with your pelvis from side to side. Remember to keep the rest of your body as still as possible. Your pelvis should be doing the work without any help from your legs or shoulders. A few inches of movement is all that is needed to get the job done.

2. You can stop for a beat when you get to the center, or, if you're comfortable with it, you can make the side-to-side motion one continuous move, stopping for a beat at the left and the right.

3. Repeat for a set of ten.

Now make pelvic circles.

1. Assume the position: Sit up straight on your ball, hands on knees, tummy tight, feet solidly planted a foot apart.

2. Start by rolling your pelvis forward. Now, roll *slowly* to the right, keeping your circle small and tight. Remember to **breathe**. Here's a visualization you won't soon forget that will help you with this exercise: Imagine that you are gripping a paintbrush between your cheeks and that you're painting circles with the brush (it's a wacky image, but it really works).

3. Go clockwise ten times. Relax. Release the muscles. Breathe.

4. Now make ten counter-clockwise circles.

5. Keep your upper body quiet and your tummy tight. Remember your paintbrush and don't forget to breathe!

Move Those Hips!

Another fun and inexpensive way to isolate and exercise your pelvic area is with an old-fashioned hula hoop! I prefer the ball exercises overall because you are more likely to do them for a longer period of time and are less likely to pull a muscle doing them! But as an adjunct to the exercise ball, the hula hoop is a hoot!

You can do the ball exercises while you watch TV, listen to music, or work at your computer answering e-mail! All it takes is a *consistent* ten or fifteen minutes a day for you to notice a difference in your level of fitness very quickly. So do your exercises without fail, because Bad Girls have swivel hips!

Speaking of swivel hips, I want to share a personal story with you that I am rather proud of. Hopefully, it will give you some additional motivation to take these exercises as seriously as I take them, and to make them part of your daily exercise routine.

When I was in graduate school, and still under supervision as a college instructor, my advisor at the time (who is a nationally known and highly regarded expert in nonverbal communication) asked the students a very pointed question about body language. He asked them to consider all of the instructors they had at the university and to name who among them had the best body language. Now, I grant you, my competition wasn't exactly stiff. However, it was still quite gratifying when a majority agreed that it was I, yours truly, who had the best body language. When pressed for more detail, several students, including female students, said *they liked the way I swiveled my hips!* I guess you never know what you're going to learn in grad school! Case closed on *that* one.

Walking at the Speed Of Sex

Taking your pelvis out of the deep freeze and giving it a life is the first step toward changing your walk forever. The second step involves learning how to use that pelvis to help you walk at a speed that spells S-E-X.

Walking at the speed of sex. It's an interesting concept, isn't it? By the time we've finished this chapter, it's a concept that is going to be an organizing principle in your Bad Girl consciousness. Because every Bad Girl I know walks at the speed of sex.

Earlier in this chapter I touched on the phenomenon of becoming *less* visible by walking fast so you already know that walking too fast isn't very sexy. What, then, is the speed of sex? Does walking at the speed of sex mean that you've got to walk slow, slow, slow? Not necessarily. There is a kind of slow that isn't particularly sexy either (a lot of Ms. Trees fall into that trap). Then what *is* the speed of sex? Before I give you a complete answer to that question, let's do a little speed check.

If you walk so fast that you would go flying off into the bushes if someone stuck their foot out in front of you, you're walking way too fast. If you walk so fast you can't feel your heels make solid contact with the ground, you walk too fast. If you walk so fast that you're always concentrating on the *next* step, not the step you're taking at that moment, you walk too fast. On the other hand, if you walk so slowly that you are always several paces behind your partner, friend, or pet turtle, you walk too slow. If you walk so slowly that you feel you have no purpose, you walk too slow. If you walk so slowly that people are shoving you out of the way, you walk too slow. If you walk so slowly that your feet sink into the mud, you walk too slow. If you walk so slowly that you can feel your energy draining, you walk too slow. If you walk so slowly that you're putting yourself to sleep, you walk way too slow.

Your Walk Is a Photo Opportunity

Here's the deal in a nutshell: *It doesn't matter how much pelvic control you have if you don't have control over your "gas pedal."* Just as flying faster than the speed of sound creates a sonic boom and the sudden expansion of air after lightning strikes creates thunder, the right walk at the right speed creates an explosive context for sex.

You've probably heard of pheromones, the body's natural chemical scents that both men and women produce and which are credited for helping to attract the opposite sex. Well, your walk can be an enhancement of that chemical "calling card," and another big piece of that potent Bad Girl package we are busy putting together.

As you might imagine, if you're whizzing by at the speed of sound yourself, there isn't a man alive who could even get a whiff of you, not to mention have enough time to take in your walk. **A man needs time to take a picture of you** (a mental picture, of course) in order to even begin to decide if he is attracted to you or not. If you're walking too fast, you're just going to be a blur with no distinct features, attributes or sexual qualities. I've said it before and I'll say it again: Walking too fast says that you're too busy to be bothered. It doesn't allow for a first impression and it doesn't allow a man time to make a sexual connection with you.

So what is wrong with *slow*? If fast is bad, why isn't slow good? It certainly gives a man time to take that picture. This is true. But here's the problem with slow: *Too* slow doesn't entice either.

Too slow gives the impression that you are aimless, not focused, tired, and with no discernible purpose. A Bad Girl *always* has a purpose. She *knows* where she's going. She knows *exactly* where she's going. She isn't rushing like a bat out of hell, but she isn't walking around with her head in the clouds, either. If walking too fast says, "Don't bother me, I'm busy," walking too slow says, "All are welcome; my time is your time." This can invite attention from men who are attracted to easy marks and I know you don't want that.

What does your internal speedometer read as you move through your life on a daily basis? Are you living life in the fastest lane? Are you dragging up the rear? Experience tells me that your walk usually gives you away.

If you walk too fast, chances are

- You drive so fast you could wallpaper your guest bathroom with speeding tickets.
- You talk so fast people think you're speaking a foreign language.
- You eat so fast you're starting on lunch at breakfast!

If you walk too slowly, you probably

- Could identify all of your friends in a line-up just from their rear ends
- Speak so slowly that people are always finishing your sentences for you
- Eat so slowly that you are just finishing your salad when everyone else is at the valet stand retrieving their cars!

Yes, I'm trying to have fun here, but I am also trying to accomplish something else. I am giving you all of these amusing images to get you to stop for a moment and take a fresh look at yourself and the speed at which you move through your life. I want you to see how your default speed (I won't call it your natural speed because I'm not so sure it *is* natural) might impact on many areas of your life—areas you may not be paying any attention to. Can you see some areas in your life in which your personal speed might be working against you?

A Bad Girl is in control of her speed. The speed at which she walks, but also much more: She is in control of the speed at which she lives her life. To have that control, she knows that she must always be working to stay fully connected to her body—all parts, not just one particular part. And that connection keeps her focus where it needs to be: on her sexual *center*, her *core*, her *essence*. It starts with a walk, but it evolves into a way of being in the world. The *walk* is just the beginning. A perfect beginning. And it's time you mastered that beginning.

You've done your work, now comes the reward. In the following exercise, I'm going to show you how to change your walk forever. Just by shifting your focus, your walk is going to go from being a boring, uneventful way of getting from point A to point B, to being a thing of beauty, poetry in motion, and a unique signature of your Bad Girl style.

You've prepared all of the necessary ingredients for your Bad Girl walk by taking control of your pelvis and tuning into the speed of sex; now it's time to take those ingredients and turn them into one delicious dish! If you're ready to learn how to walk on the wild side, read on!

exercise 3:

Walking "The Walk"

If your videotape buddy is still available, I would definitely videotape this exercise for comparison's sake. You'll be amazed at the difference!

1. Stand with your arms relaxed at your sides. Breathe deeply into your solar plexus. Loosen your head and neck by doing a few head rolls. Get rid of any tension in your limbs by giving them a vigorous shake.

2. Begin walking. Ask you walk—

3. **Imagine that you are being pulled forward by a string attached to your pelvic area (your groin).**

4. Keep your attention focused on your pelvis as you walk. Keep your abdomen lightly contracted.

5. Notice how by keeping your focus on your lower torso area as you walk, you are walking at a lovely pace; not too fast, not too slow, just right. **That speed is the speed of sex.**

Walking at the speed of sex is achieved through the combination of keeping your *mental* and *physical* focus on your lower torso as you walk, sit, and stand. I have never known this particular one-two punch not to have a remarkable effect on the way a woman looks and feels as she makes her way through the world. Practice sitting on a chair or sofa with your focus remaining on your pelvic area. You should find that you even sit and stand differently when your focus remains where it should.

As you continue to walk, can you sense how your spine has fallen into alignment? Can you see how your arms are now swinging naturally at your sides? Can you feel how beautifully your hips are now swinging from side to side? Can you believe how incredibly *sexy* it feels to walk this way? It is impossible to slump, slouch, or revert to your old way of walking if you consciously remind yourself to *lead with your pelvis* as you walk. You are training yourself to *switch your focus*; a very valuable skill that we'll explore, expand on, and develop even more in the next chapter.

Another gigantic benefit of keeping your focus on your pelvic area as you walk, sit, and stand, is the constant *psychological* and *physiological* connection to your sexuality you create and maintain. In fact, you might want to imagine the string that is pulling your pelvis forward as being your constant invisible connection to your sexuality. It's a thought that will put a definite twinkle in your eye and a little "I've got a secret" smile on your lips.

It feels so incredibly good to walk this way that it will quickly become second nature to you. When your friends, family, or co-workers ask you about the change in the way you are walking (and they will definitely notice a change), just tell them that you have been working out—which is true, of course. You are under no obligation whatsoever to tell *anyone* that you are being led from the pelvis by an invisible string that keeps you in constant connection to your sexual source. And whatever you do, don't even *think* about telling Mr. Wonderful (who suddenly wants to jump your bones, for reasons he doesn't understand). It's *your* little secret. Having little secrets like this is what being Bad is all about. If you are walking the Bad Girl walk right now, your little secret is already shaking things up, in the Baddest possible way.

Chapter 5

Bad Girls Know How to Talk Sexy, In and Out of Bed

*J*enna has a problem that lots of Good Girls have. When she *thinks* about sex she thinks in hard-core XXX, but when she opens her mouth and tries to ask her lover for what she wants or tell him how she feels during sex, her words come out PG-13. Jenna's idea of talking dirty is saying, "I want to make love." Saying the word "penis" makes her blush. Saying any sexy four-letter words is simply out of the question. And when she is having sex, she moans on occasion, but otherwise it's so quiet you could hear a pin drop.

Good Girls have a problem with their vocabulary skills that gets in the way of a hot encounter. When it comes to the subject of sex, they tend to believe that silence is golden and they follow this rule even more closely once the lovemaking starts. When we go to the movies and we see a love scene, often the only thing we can hear is the music from the soundtrack. But in real life that kind of hushed silence gets a little boring after five or ten minutes with a flesh and blood partner.

The Good Girl's Guide to Bad Girl Sex

Whether it's during seduction or during great sex, Bad Girls have vocabulary skills that can't be learned in any classroom (except for mine, of course!). Their ability to say just the right words at the right time is something to marvel at. They can heat up a room with a single sentence. They even *breathe* sexy. What they *don't* do is waste their words on uninteresting small talk that ruins a mood.

In this chapter, you're going to learn how Bad Girls talk to the men they desire. You're going to learn when to talk and when not to talk, what to say, and how to say it. But most importantly, you're going to learn how sexy saying these special words can make you and your partner feel.

Bad Girls Use the "V" Word to Their Advantage

Here's a riddle for you: What is something you use everyday, never give a second thought, but would miss terribly if it went away? I'll give you a hint: It begins with a "v." No, it's not *that* "v" word. The answer is: your **voice**. What does your voice have to do with being a sexy Bad Girl? Absolutely *everything*.

Lauren Bacall. Marilyn Monroe. Greta Garbo. Besides being legendary sex symbols, the other thing all of these screen divas have in common is that they all have unforgettable sexy voices. In fact, I'm hard pressed to think of any well-known sex symbol who *doesn't* have a sexy voice. Not surprisingly, all three of the actresses mentioned above could also sing. The reason it isn't surprising is because it takes breath control to sing and it's impossible to have a sexy voice without having control over your breath.

When "talkies," or movies with sound, were first introduced, many film actresses feared for their careers—and rightly so. For as it turned out, many of the greatest silent film stars had voices that shattered their sex-symbol persona—squeaky voices, childish voices, grating voices, voices only their mothers could love (and *they* might've been lying, too!). You can look like a dream, but if you open your mouth and the sound that comes out makes people want to duck and cover, your life can seem more like a nightmare.

Breath Control

Changing the way you breathe can have an amazing effect on your voice. Most people don't ever think about the way that they breathe. It's going to happen whether they think about it or not, so what's the big deal, right? The truth of the matter is, with a little thought and a little practice, you can learn how to use your breath to do a lot more than simply get you from one day to the next.

Conscious breathing can simultaneously relax and energize you. It's hard to be Bad when you're feeling jittery, tired, and deflated. Not breathing fully traps energy in your body. So if you're nervous, for instance, not breathing fully only makes you *more* nervous. **Bad Girls breathe fully**.

Deer caught in the headlights, possums who sense danger, and women on a first date all have something in common: They tend to quit breathing. Let's say you're having dinner with a man you've had your eye on for some time and you're feeling a bit nervous. Chances are you're taking short, shallow breaths, which is common when people are experiencing stress. The fact that you're not taking *relaxed, deep, slow* (very sexy) breaths, *will* register with your date. It may not register *consciously* with him, but it will register somewhere; and it may leave him with the impression that you are apprehensive, jumpy, and not particularly fun to be around. None of this is terribly sexy.

Consciously and consistently catching your breath will calm your nerves, recharge your internal battery, and provide a solid foundation from which you can be your most Bad. When you combine conscious breathing with the voice-centering techniques you're also going to learn in this chapter, you have the key to developing your own unforgettable, red hot, *sexy*, Bad Girl voice.

exercise 1:

Conscious Breathing

1. Lie on your back.

2. Exhale through your mouth, completely emptying the lungs of air.

3. As you inhale through your nostrils (not your mouth), imagine *lowering* (not raising) your diaphragm, and allow the air to enter your lungs.

4. Feel your abdomen slowly expand with air, filling the bottom of the lungs.

5. As the air rises, filling your lungs and gently expanding your ribcage, top off your inhalation and let the lungs completely fill with air by allowing the air to gently *lift* the collar bones.

6. Now exhale fully through the mouth.

7. Repeat the process for several minutes. In through the nose, deep, deep, deep, then out through the mouth.

Things to keep in mind as you do the exercise:

- Keep your breathing smooth and easy; no need to force, gasp, or gulp.

- Don't try to stifle the sound.

- In order to enjoy maximum rejuvenating benefits, keep your mind completely focused on the action of the breath.

- Practice makes perfect; it's normal for this way of breathing to feel a little strange at first, but once you see how much better it can make you feel, you will be inspired to practice it daily.

As you become more used to conscious breathing, you won't need to lie down in order to practice it. In fact, the goal is to integrate Conscious Breathing seamlessly into your "walking" life.

Healthy human lungs are capable of holding four quarts of air. The average person only inhales half a quart of air in a typical breath. That's only 12 percent of what we're capable of! Conscious Breathing will give your body more oxygen with which to operate, your brain more oxygen with which to think, and your voice more power to be Bad, Bad, Bad.

Using Your Voice to Create a Consistent Message

Now that your lungs have at least double the amount of air to work with on a regular basis, you have the lung support that you need to begin developing the voice that you truly deserve.

I mentioned her once before, but she's worth mentioning again, as Audrey Hepburn's Eliza Doolittle in *My Fair Lady* provides a wonderful example of the importance of a woman's speech and voice (and if you haven't ever seen *My Fair Lady*, rent it for a delightful treat!). When Professor Higgins first meets Eliza Doolittle, she is a guttersnipe with a voice to match: nasal, sharp, and shrewish. After she goes through her transformation ("The rain in Spain falls mainly on the plain . . ."), her new voice and speech are in many ways even more enchanting than her new looks.

Here's another example to consider. What if the Mona Lisa suddenly came to life and opened her mouth to speak? For centuries she has been celebrated as one of the most beautiful, mysterious, and sensuous women ever immortalized on canvas. When you look at the Mona Lisa, it's easy to imagine her as being soft-spoken, with a low voice that is demure, sexy, and inviting, don't you agree? Can you imagine the shock and the disappointment people would experience if the Mona Lisa could speak, but she sounded like Carla from the TV show *Cheers*? Or the nosy neighbor Mrs. Kravitz from the '60s show *Bewitched*?

Well, I hate to be the one to tell you this, but that is exactly the kind of cognitive dissonance that many women are creating for their male audience when they open their mouths and start to speak. Cognitive dissonance is one of those $500 academic phrases that really isn't terribly complex. Simply put, cognitive dissonance is created when a piece of knowledge someone believes to be true is contradicted by a new piece of evidence that cannot be ignored.

Here's a hypothetical example for you: Let's say you're at the market buying groceries. You're in the produce section thumping melons for ripeness when suddenly you spy Mr. GQ near the leafy greens. This guy looks like a model who just escaped from a runway in Paris. *Everything* is j-u-s-t so: clean, elegant, and stylish. Suddenly, you develop an urgent need for lettuce, so you navigate your cart closer to the Armani-clad vision. You're just wheeling up beside him, so close you can almost smell him, when he turns your way and opens his mouth as though he's about to speak. You're ecstatic! You can barely breathe! But instead of hearing, "My God, you're beautiful. Would you like to have dinner with me tonight?," Mr. Wonderful parts his lips and lets out a belch so loud and long it wilts the parsley in his hand. That feeling you have? That feeling of your mind being blown? *That* is cognitive dissonance.

An ear-splitting belch coming from a handsome, well-groomed man (especially in a public place!) sends an *inconsistent message* and that creates cognitive dissonance. What would *you* do in the scenario I described above? How would you deal with this contradiction? Wouldn't you turn on your heel and run in the other direction? I know I probably would.

But now back to you. You don't have to belch in public to turn a guy off (though that certainly is one way to do it). You might not be aware of it, but if your voice and your language are not *consistent* with the rest of the picture you're presenting to the world, you may be driving people away from you in your personal life. You might even be robbing yourself of all the success you could be having in your *professional* life. In chapters one through four of this book, you learned the secrets to dressing, looking, and walking like a Bad Girl. But in order to present a *completely consistent message*—a 100 percent Bad Girl Message—that doesn't confuse your audience and subsequently drive them away, it is essential that you learn to *speak* like a serious Bad Girl, too.

Bad Girls Know How to Talk Sexy

Verbal Control

There are three basic parts to speech:

1. What you say (words)
2. How you say it (tone)
3. How you sound (vocal qualities)

Having mastery over these three basic parts is a Bad Girl's mark of distinction, as well as a badge of honor. And it isn't all that hard to accomplish. How do you start? Just as you had to study the way that you walked before you could change it, you have to really *hear* the way that you talk before you can change that, too. So let's get right to it!

Every time I assign this next exercise in my class, some students express concern that videotaping themselves talking will make them forever more self-conscious and uncomfortable with their own voice and language. But experience tells me that the fear these women express is really based on their internal hunch that when it comes to language and voice, they are somewhat careless, sloppy, and *un*sexy. I tell these students what I'm about to tell you: videotaping yourself speaking and having the courage to view that tape and learn from that tape, will, vocally speaking, actually make you far more natural, self-confident, and in control. The change will happen very quickly. Not only will you be "ready for your close-up" and therefore more attractive to men, but you will find your professional life benefiting from your efforts as well.

exercise 2:

Tape Yourself Talking

A video camera is preferable, but you can also use a tape recorder for this exercise.

1. Invite your camera buddy over for lunch or dinner. Besides having earned a free meal from you (don't you agree?), their job this time is simply to provide conversation.

2. Set up the video camera in such a way that it will tape the two of you as you eat your meal. If you're using a tape recorder, place it on the table beside you and do a test to make sure that it is working. Be sure to use at least a 90-minute tape, so that if you forget to flip it over, you will still have recorded a lengthy portion of yourself talking.

3. If you tend not to be particularly talkative, have a couple of stories in mind that you can tell. This exercise won't work if you don't talk!

4. Grab a pen and a pad of paper. To complete this exercise, you are going to **watch and/or listen to your tape a total of *three times.***

5. **The First Time:** *Listen to the words you use.* What are you saying? Do you use words such as: "like," "you know," "um," "uh," and "really," over and over again in your conversation? Incessant use of this kind of verbal filler can give your listener the impression that you are either: (a) immature, (b) not particularly well educated, or (c) linguistically lazy. No good choices there! Remember when California's Valley Girls became a national joke? Their way of speaking was a source of amusement for the whole country. Who could forget: "Like, fer

sure!," "Gag me with a spoon!," "As if!," and so on. A few colloquialisms now and then are fine, but when they become the very foundation of your speech, it's time to take back control.
Bad Girls watch their mouths.

6. **The Second Time:** *Listen to the tone of voice you use.* Does your tone of voice match the words you're saying? For instance, when you ask a question, do you sound genuinely interested, or do you sound bored? Do you sound like you already know what the answer should be (subtly steering the conversation)? When you answer a question, do you sound forthcoming? Or defensive? You can be saying all the right things, but if you're not saying them with the right tone of voice, your well-chosen words will not have the effect you want them to.
Bad Girls watch how they say things.

7. **The Third Time:** *Listen to your voice.* What does your voice sound like? Is it pleasant to listen to? Where does it sound like your voice is projecting from? Does it sound like it's coming from your head (nasal)? Your throat (hoarse or flat)? Do you talk in a little baby voice? Or maybe you sound harsh. It's not possible to completely change the nature of your voice, but there are steps you can take to change certain vocal qualities. If your voice sounds like music to *your* ears, it will sound that way to others, too.
Bad Girls sound good.

Congratulations on being brave enough to take such an honest look at yourself. Your desire to be Bad is a really beautiful thing! You now have a lot of information about what you say, how you say it, and how you sound. Were there any surprises in it for you? Use index cards or your notebook to jot down your observations while they're still fresh in your mind. It will help to have these notes for easy reference (and reminders) later.

Listen Up!

You've already accomplished a lot, but I want to make sure we cover all of the bases here, and one that is easily missed is *listening skills*. You've taken a hard look at the words you used on your tape, but how were your listening skills during this last exercise? Did you give your friend an opportunity to talk? Did you let her/him finish her/his sentences without interrupting? There's a secret to coming across as absolutely fascinating to men. Want to know what it is? **Listen to them**. It's that simple. Instead of getting lost in your own thoughts and your own words, listen well, listen constantly, and periodically ask questions that show how well you've been listening—questions about what they think, what they do, what they like, what they like about what they do.

The more you listen and ask questions, the more attractive, mysterious, and intriguing you will become. Then, when you finally do say more than a sentence or two, the man you've been listening to will be completely turned on by the sound of your voice and hungry to learn all he can about you. If the guy *doesn't* ever turn the tables and ask you about yourself, you will know early on that you're probably dealing with someone who is, shall we say, "self-involved," and you can make your next move accordingly. This listening technique isn't just for a dating scenario; it works equally well with clients, bosses, children, lovers, husbands . . . you name it.

And what about swearing? Has it become a habit for you? Do you make sailors blush? Although swearing has reached "epidemic" proportions in the U.S., you never know when someone you're talking to might find it offensive. If that "someone" is with you on date (or, heaven forbid, interviewing you for a job), you've pretty much just blown yourself out of the water. I often think about swearing the way I think about fine art: You have to prove that you can paint classically before you are taken seriously as an abstract artist, and you have to gain your listener's respect by speaking "classically" before risking "jazzing up" your speech with an epithet.

If swearing has become a habit for you, make a commitment to consciously abstain from using swear words for one week. You'll be amazed at how much more of your vocabulary you will use. I'm not talking about sexy language here—there's a time and place for that in your romantic vocabulary and we'll get to this very soon. No, I'm talking about language that cheapens you—sailor's language, as my grandmother used to say. There's nothing sexy or Bad about cheap talk.

Vocal Control

You have learned how to control your breath through conscious breathing, and you know how to control your words through conscious speaking (and listening), but how do you control your voice? The right words will be lost if they are delivered in a nasal honk that curls the hair of your listener. Are there steps you can take to turn your goose-like honk or your Minnie Mouse squeak into an Eartha Kitt purr? Well, yes, there are steps you can take, and no, it may not produce a miracle. But using the same focus and visualization techniques you have already used to walk the Bad Girl walk can help you *sound* more like the Bad Girl you really are. All it takes, really, is a shift in your focus.

Vocal Centering

Some people speak from their heads, which produces a high-pitched voice. Others speak through their noses, which gives their voices a nasal twang. Still others speak from the throat, but stay disconnected from the rest of their body, giving the voice some hoarseness, perhaps, but no real depth. Just as a singer cannot produce or sustain a pleasant sounding note by projecting from the head, nose, or throat, none of these are the optimum place from which to project a Bad Girl voice.

To walk the Bad Girl walk, you placed your focus on your pelvis and you imagined your walk as originating from that place. To get your voice out of your head, nose, or throat, and consequently produce more resonant, sexy tones, you similarly place your focus on a centering spot on your body, and in this case, that centering place is your *diaphragm*.

Your diaphragm is located in the middle of your chest, about two inches below the spot right between your breasts (the bottom of your ribcage). Place your hand there now. Feel your belly rising and falling. Feel your heart beating.

After a few moments, you may start to feel soothed; a sense of comfort and healing may wash over you. When I am stressed out or upset,

I place my hand over my diaphragm, close my eyes, take a conscious breath, and allow the sense of connection and groundedness to renew and calm me. Something else remarkable happens when I do this: **When I consciously center myself in my diaphragm, my voice drops down into my chest and I begin speaking from this place**.

If I had previously been speaking excitedly, with my voice creeping up in pitch until it sounded as though it was emanating from around my ears somewhere, *centering myself in my diaphragm* brings my voice back down into "Eartha Kitt" territory. This "chest centering" will also put the brakes on your w.p.m. (words per minute) if you have been talking at supersonic speeds.

If you only learn to do *one thing* in this whole book, learn to do this.

- **THIS** is the place you want to come from to be the genuine article.
- **THIS** is the place you go to, to connect with yourself.
- **THIS** is the place where Bad—in the *best* sense—resides.

Here's an exercise that will help you coax your voice down out of the rafters and into the very seat of your most grounded, authentic self.

---

exercise 3:
Finding Your Bad Girl Voice

Every voice is unique. Your Bad Girl voice isn't going to sound exactly like any one else's. This exercise isn't about trying to force yourself to sound like someone else, or doing an imitation of someone else. The goal of this exercise is to help liberate the voice that is already within you, just waiting to be discovered.

1. Sit comfortably with your feet flat on the ground and your back straight.

2. Place your hand (palm down) on your diaphragm. Nestle it well between your breasts. Don't cup your hand; make sure it is lying flat against your body.

---

3. Take several conscious breaths (in through the nose). Let the air fill your abdomen and also rise to the top of your head—the deepest kind of breath. Exhale through your mouth. Keep your hand on your diaphragm.

4. Inhale once again. On the exhalation, *begin a high-pitched hum.* You are going to start at "high C" on the scale, and run down one octave. Imagine the hum starting at the top of your head. As your pitch descends the tonal scale, imagine it also descending through your head, so that when your exhalation is depleted, the hum has come to rest in your nasal cavity.

5. Breathe in. On this next exhalation, *imagine the hum originating from your nasal cavity* (instead of the top of your head). Begin the tone at "middle C," and run down another octave. This time, when you run out of breath, imagine the hum coming to rest in your throat.

6. On your third and final exhalation, *begin the hum where you left off last time: same location* (throat), *same pitch* (the lowest note). During this exhalation, as your hum descends the tonal scale, *picture your voice literally dropping down through your chest cavity. Let it drop.* By the time your breath finally runs out, you should feel as though your voice has come to rest *in your diaphragm*, right next to where your hand is nestled.

   That final note that ends up resting against your hand—that note from low in the center of your chest—is *your* Bad Girl Voice.

Try reading the sentence above out loud from that place you have just discovered. Imagine your voice, your power, and your truth as being nestled there, between and slightly beneath your breasts. *Project* from that place. *Own it.* It is *yours* to use, enjoy, and revel in. You will probably need to practice the humming exercise for a while to help remind you of where your true voice is and how to access it. After a while, if you hear your voice sliding up the scale, all you will have to do is picture it coming from your diaphragm, and it will drop back down. Then you'll be right back where you belong: centered, powerful, and BAD.

Are You Ready to Talk Sexy?

There is a reason I have led you through all of the previous vocal exercises in this chapter before arriving at our final destination: talking sexy. I'm sure you will agree that it was necessary to get you grounded and centered in a place of power and awareness before embarking on a journey that will require all of that from you, and more. In order to make your words like little firebombs that ignite upon contact with your lover's ears, those words have to be *connected* to something, or else the effect may very well have an almost comical overtone.

I wrote an entire book on this subject called *Talk Sexy to the One You Love*, so this is obviously something that is near and dear to my heart. Of all of the techniques, positions, lotions, and potions that I know of, use, and recommend to others, the most important, most transforming, and most powerful aphrodisiac of them all, by far, is learning how to talk sexy in a genuine and convincing manner. When your lovemaking comes from a connection that is forged from words that spring from your most intimate and erotic thoughts, fantasies, and desires, you are in Bad Girl flow, and your natural creativity is being given full expression. It's when we stifle these words that the "disconnect" occurs and we find ourselves feeling less than satisfied. But you're not the same woman you were four chapters ago, and you have everything you need to make talking sexy a reality in your life.

What's That You Say?

What are the sexual words, phrases, and requests that rattle around in your head that you are too shy, scared, or embarrassed to say to your man? I don't just mean when you are actually having sex, but also those down and dirty thoughts that pop into your mind at the most ordinary times, like when you're strolling down the street hand in hand, having dinner at a restaurant, or sitting on the sofa watching the evening news. Those words that come into your mind organically and naturally are your future sex life's best friends. It's time to bring those friends in from the cold!

I wouldn't be surprised if some of you are so good at pushing those thoughts away that you are telling yourself that you don't *have* those kind of thoughts. To that, I say . . . bull-loney! You most certainly do! They may just be so faint that you can barely hear them, and so ephemeral that they evaporate like last night's dream, but they are there. And we're going to turn those whispers into screams, if need be, so that you can hear them, embrace them, and put them to work for you.

exercise 4:
Fishing for Words (Part 1)

This exercise involves fantasy, imagination, and visualization. Allow yourself a half hour or more to complete it. If you live with someone, pick a time when they're not home; in order to relax completely, you need to know you won't be disturbed. Is there a particular singer or album that puts you in a sexy mood? Feel free to play it (softly) while you have fun with this very enjoyable exercise. Have your Bad Girl journal or a pad of paper close by.

1. Lie on your back on your bed, sofa, or sheepskin rug in front of the fireplace (if you're so lucky). Take a few deep, cleansing breaths. Close your eyes.

2. Picture yourself in a private place with your lover, or with anyone else that turns you on (this is *your* fantasy and there are no wrongs). Where are you in your fantasy? Are you in bed? In the back seat of a car? On the kitchen table? Pick a spot that makes you *sizzle*.

3. Your man looks *hot*. He's wearing a black T-shirt that really shows off his biceps/pecs/abs (whatever turns you on the most). As you look at him, what thoughts are you having? Imagine yourself telling your lover the thoughts that are in your head.
   • **See** yourself sharing your thoughts with your lover.
   • **Hear** yourself saying the words that you are feeling.
   • **Feel** the words coming from your diaphragm and your connection to them.

4. His arm feels good around your shoulders. He's wearing your favorite aftershave and smells good enough to eat. In fact, you start to nibble on his ear. As you slide the smooth lobe gently into your mouth, your desire begins to mount. Physiological changes are beginning to occur: Your clitoris is getting hard, you can feel yourself getting wet, your nipples are aching to be touched.
   - **See** yourself telling your lover what your body is doing.
   - **Hear** yourself asking your lover for what you want.
   - **Feel** the connection you have to those words.

Since this is *your* fantasy, I will bow out now and let you take over from here. Try to take your fantasy all the way through the lovemaking experience. Continue *seeing* yourself speaking the words you are thinking. *Hear* yourself. *Feel* the words coming from your centered place.

Please keep in mind that the scenario above is just a suggestion; if you prefer your guy in leather, in a business suit, or in his birthday suit, have at it. The most important thing is that it's a fantasy that works for *you*.

Feeling horny right now? You're not alone. A lot of women report the need to masturbate during and/or after this exercise (if you felt the need to masturbate *before* the exercise, more power to you!). *Use your aroused state to propel yourself into another fantasy.* Make it different this time. Are there any everyday activities you do that put you in a sexual state of mind? Let your imagination go there now.

What Really *Happens in Bed?*

I had one client, Heather, who overheated (sexually speaking) whenever she and her man were putting clean sheets on the bed. For the longest time she would push her thoughts and feelings aside because she felt it was weird to become aroused during such a mundane chore. The warmth and fresh smell of the sheets, the connection she felt with her partner as they worked together to prepare their bed, the physical movement; all of these things contributed to filling her with desire. It wasn't until Heather did the exercise above that she was able to put into words what she was feeling. First, she got to practice putting her thoughts into words in the privacy of her own mind. Then, she got to *see* herself communicating her thoughts and desires to her lover with connection and confidence. Third, she got to imagine her words producing a positive outcome, culminating in a satisfying sexual encounter with her lover. Confident of what she would say, how she would say it, and of her actions having a positive outcome, Heather was able to re-enact her visualization in actuality the next time she and her lover made the bed together. She later told me that it was very possibly the best sex she had ever had. Needless to say, she became a big fan of the visualization technique and employed it often!

Does that story spark any recollections for you? Are there any triggers in your day when you find yourself getting aroused for no apparent reason? For instance, do you come home from your aerobics class ready for love? Do you want to pounce on your man ever time he mows the lawn? These times are gifts that should be coaxed out of the shadows and into the light. Allow yourself to have a full-blown fantasy involving whatever that activity happens to be. See yourself putting your thoughts and desires into words like Heather did. Visualize the positive outcome your words will produce. Enjoy the fantasy.

exercise 5:
Fishing for Words (Part 2)

The first part of this exercise involved visualization and imagination. And because visualizations are similar to dreams and you are apt to forget them if you don't write them down, the second part of this exercise involves committing the words you used in your visualizations to paper.

In the paragraphs that follow, I am going to ask you a series of questions. Please rewrite the questions in your journal and give yourself plenty of room to answer them.

Copy and complete:

1. In what ways did you express yourself in your fantasies that you don't express yourself in waking life? For instance, did you ask for what you want? Or tell your lover what you want to do to him? Did you compliment your lover's body parts or describe your own physical sensations?

2. How did expressing yourself in that way make you feel?

3. What words and phrases did you say in your fantasy that you don't use or say in your waking life?

4. How did using those words make you feel?

5. Did you use any words or phrases that made you uncomfortable? If so, why?

6. Which words and phrases did you most enjoy saying?

7. Were you surprised by anything you did or said in your fantasies?

Barbara's (B)ad-Libs

The whole thrust of this book has really been about getting to know who you are when you emerge from the shadows and step fully into your womanhood. I'm hoping that during Fishing for Words, you saw and heard a side of yourself that was new and exciting to you.

We already know the immense power your visualizations have. They were indispensable in your discovery and development of your Bad Girl wardrobe. Now , with the help of one of my very favorite exercises, you will use the rich material your fantasies have given you to create your very own Bad Girl vocabulary.

Bad Girls Know How to Talk Sexy

Did you ever go to summer camp? One of my fondest memories is when the lights in our cabin would go out and a dozen twelve- to fourteen-year-old girls would play "Mad-Libs" in the dark. Mad-Libs (a take off on ad-libs) involved fill-in-the-blank stories that revolved around a theme that wasn't revealed until after all of the blanks had been filled in. The most fun occurred when one of the nouns or adjectives created a "blue" Mad-Lib; we would laugh so hard and out of control, our counselor would come in and threaten us with kitchen duty for a week if we didn't quiet down.

It's time to play this ad-lib game again, but a much more adult version. This time the theme is S-E-X, and the blanks are going to be filled in with the words and phrases that you wrote down from the previous exercise.

(B)ad Lib #1: A Letter To Your Lover

Here's a great way to introduce your new vocabulary to your lover (and warm up your engine at the same time). Just imagine how thrilled he'll be to find this letter waiting for him on his pillow!

> *Darling. I've been thinking about you all day and about how much I love your (noun). I can't get it out of my head. I love the way it feels in my (noun). Just thinking about it there makes my (noun) (adjective). I wish you were here right now so that I could run my (noun) up and down your (noun). No one's (noun) has ever affected me the way yours does. The way you (verb) me with it makes me want to scream with delight. My (noun) is (verb)-ing just imagining you (verb)-ing me. Come and get me, darling. My (noun) is your (noun).*

How's that for some big-time fun? Ready for another one? Try this one on for size.

Bad Girls Know How to Talk Sexy

(B)ad Lib #2: The Bad Dinner

This is definitely not a Bad-Lib for your first date! But you'll know when the time is right to use it.

> *I love to eat* (noun) *because it's such a sensual food. The way it feels on my tongue reminds me of* (verb)-*ing you because it's so soft and smooth. I know they say that oysters are an aphrodisiac, but for me,* (noun) *really puts me in the mood. The combination of the texture, the smell, and the taste excite my senses to such a degree that I get completely turned on. So much so that right now, as I sit here, I wish I could come over there, sit on your lap, and slip my* (noun) *down your* (noun). *I'd like to take this olive oil and drizzle it on your* (noun) *and then use my hand to* (verb) *you until you're close to* (verb)-*ing. Then I'd take the whipped cream from my cappucino, smear it on my* (noun), *and hide you under the table while you* (verb) *it off me. And when neither of us could stand it any more, I'd let you take me right here on this banquette, and slide your olive-oiled* (noun) *into my* (adjective), (adjective) (noun), *until we both* (verb) *like we've never* (verb)-*ed before.*

If you even get through half of that Bad-Lib before he's yelling for the check, I'll be amazed! Unless he's too mesmerized to move, of course. As with all of these verbal exercises, the key to using them successfully is making them your own and using words and phrases that feel right *for you*. Remember, you're not imitating anyone or anything; be as genuine as you can be. Obviously, don't *say* it if you don't *mean* it! If you don't intend to have sexual relations with someone, don't Bad-Lib them! That could only lead to much confusion, or worse. Although Bad-Libs are extremely playful, it isn't a game that you are playing, it's the real deal. Bad-Libs should only be used when you intend to carry through with what you are proposing.

Bad Girls Know How to Talk Sexy

(B)ad Lib #3: Bad in Bed

Finally. The main event. What all of the deep breathing, humming, and visualization have been preparing you for: how to talk Bad in bed. Here's how you can take a few glowing coals and fan them until they're a raging bonfire of desire, emotion, and physical passion. Talking sexy in bed is what separates the Bad Girls from the merely bold. Since this isn't "The Good Girl's Guide to *Bold* Girl Sex," I'm figuring you must want to be Bad. Do you? Do you want to be Bad? You do? Then wrap your lips around this one . . .

I've been thinking about your hands on my (noun) all day. Can I put your hand there myself? Your fingers are so strong. I love how their slight roughness feels against the silkiness of my (noun). I'm getting (adjective). Can you feel it? (Verb) me again; just like you just did. Do you mind if I (verb) your (noun)? I'd really like to. Actually, I need to. Actually, if I don't, I may just go out of my mind. Give it to me. Give me your (adjective) (noun). Put it in my (noun). Do you like that? I like it. I like it a lot. In fact, I love it. You're getting so (adjective). Touch my (noun). Look what you're doing to me. I'm going to (verb) my (noun) so that you can (verb) me there. Just like that. Just like that. Give me more. I need more. Touch my (noun) while you (verb) me. Feel my (noun). It feels so good. Your (noun) feels so good. Your (noun) tastes so good. Does my (noun) taste good? Tell me how good it tastes. You're driving me crazy. I'm ready for your (noun). Can I have it? Can I have it now? Oh yes. Thank you. Thank you. My (noun) is on fire. If you touch it I might . . . You're like a (noun) of (noun) inside me. I can't take much more. I'm close to (verb)-ing. (Verb) with me. I want to (verb) with you. It's close; it's so close. (Verb) me harder. Faster. Deeper. Harder.

Whew! Personally, I'm ready for a cigarette and I don't even smoke! Hot enough for you? BAD enough for you? If not, bump it up a notch or two. If it's a little too hot to handle, choose the phrases you like, use those, and then make up some of your own. This isn't a script to be memorized so much as a "blue"-print for your own personal dialogue. You don't need me to put words in your mouth; you've become quite proficient at that on your own. And you are sounding like one Bad package now, truly talking the Bad Girl talk.

Chapter 6

Bad Girls Know Their Bodies

A lot of women who want to be bad have a very complex love/hate relationship with their sexuality. Erika is a perfect example. Erika says that one of her favorite things in the entire world is performing oral sex on her lover. She can talk endlessly about the shape, size, and taste of his penis, and the way it feels inside her mouth. She loves the sight of the first "tear," as she calls it—a drop of preseminal fluid emerging from the tip. She especially loves to watch his facial expressions change as he climaxes.

So what's the problem? The problem is that Erika has very little to say about her own sexual response. Erika rarely feels very aroused—not from oral sex, not from intercourse; and she has never been able to climax with a partner. Not once. She can masturbate herself to orgasm if she is alone and doesn't feel a time constraint, but she describes her climax as "a quiet little twitch." Erika says that she loves sex because it brings her closer to her partner, but she also acknowledges that she is frustrated much of the time. She can never really feel turned on because her body doesn't seem to turn on. She can get excited about her partner, but she can't get excited about herself.

Not surprisingly, Erika's lover is also frustrated. Erika's lack of sexual response is very discouraging to him. Despite Erika's assurances that "it's not him," it also makes him feel inadequate as a lover.

Erika needs to break down some of her barriers to feeling good. Do you? **If you're going to be Bad, sex *has* to feel good.** It has to feel more than good. It has to feel great. Really fabulous. Powerful. Consuming. Memorable. If your experience of sex is just "okay," then your attitude towards sex is going to be just okay. In this chapter, we're going to work on changing the way sex feels. No more "okay." It's time for a few "WOWs."

You're going to learn steps you can take to break through some of the basic emotional and physiological blocks that keep you from having the best sex of your life. You'll also learn exercises that will heighten your erotic sensitivity, increase your sensuality, and magnify the moment-by-moment experience of arousal.

Bad Girl: Know Thyself

One of my greatest life lessons came in my early twenties, when I was in the throes of one of my first important romances. One night, in the early days of our relationship, my boyfriend and I were making love. As our passion grew, my boyfriend slid down my body and began to perform oral sex on me. It was my first time, and although it felt wonderful to me, I couldn't help feeling a bit uncomfortable. Surprisingly, the questions most on my mind were these: Was my vagina normal? Was it attractive? Was it a turn-on or a turn-off? If my boyfriend had done this with other women, which I assumed he had, how would I compare with these other women?

These thoughts flitted through my mind, almost unconsciously—I never spoke them out loud to my young lover. He was a special guy, however, because almost as though he was reading my mind, he said to me, "You have the most beautiful pussy." I do? I was flabbergasted, thrilled, incredulous, slightly embarrassed, and complimented in the extreme. Not only was he the only one ever in my whole life to say something positive about my vagina, except for my gynecologist, he was the only person in the world to ever take the time to even *look* at it; *including me*! His sincere, spontaneous, and generous compliment made me realize how little I knew about my own body. Why didn't I already know that I have a beautiful vagina? Why did I have to wait twenty-three years to discover that? What *else* was I ignorant about concerning my own body and sexuality?

Let me ask you a pointed question: How well do you know your own body? If you had to write down the recipe of the ingredients it takes to transport you from cold (not aroused) to red hot (climax state), could you do it? I don't mean in generalities, either. I'm speaking technically here; step by step, physical actions that take you from point A to point Z. What are the steps? How does it feel along the way? And how much time do you need at each step?

Since there's no way to be subtle about this, I'll just come out and say it: What about your vagina? That's right, your *vagina*. Could you identify it in a line up? Without the birthmark on your upper thigh to clue you in, just looking at an extreme close up of your private parts, would you know which one was yours? Quick—where's your G-spot? Could you insert your finger into your vagina and know just where to find it?

**A Bad Girl can answer "yes, yes, and yes"
to all of these questions . . . and *more*.**

Bad Girls don't allow themselves to remain ignorant about their own bodies. Bad Girls know themselves *inside out*. If you know exactly how your own equipment works, you won't have to depend on a foreign operator (a man) or on happenstance to show you the ropes of your own anatomy and makeup. You will know exactly how everything is strung together, how everything works, and what it takes to get your juices flowing and your temperature rising.

Map the Terrain

In this chapter, I want you to approach your body as if it's a new continent and you've been sent to learn its topography, gold mines, mountain ranges, and buried treasures. Get out your compass, because you're about to learn north from south, east from west, up from down, and your labia from your libido. You're going to learn its hot spots, its rushing rapids, and its volatile volcanoes. In other words, you're about to become an expert on *you*. It all starts with a simple . . . touch.

Fact: *very few of us get touched enough.*

Even if you are happily partnered, I will bet that you don't get stroked, caressed, bear-hugged, or massaged enough. Did you get enough touch today? What about yesterday? What about the day before? One way to put more "touch" in our lives is to *do it ourselves.* Besides just making you feel good, it's how you learn what kind of touch, on what part of your body, makes you feel *best*.

exercise 1:

Touch Yourself (Sensate Focus Touch)

It's finally time to get naked! Always one of *my* favorite times. Carve out some private moments for yourself and head for the bedroom.

The purpose of this exercise is to give your body a wake-up call and to reacclimate it to a new level of sensitivity. You're also going to track your body's reaction to touch. Here's the very simple way you're going to measure your body's response and level of arousal:

> **Level 1** = Zero to low level of arousal
> **Level 2** = Moderate level of arousal
> **Level 3** = Intense level of arousal
> **Level 4** = Orgasmic level of arousal

At each stage of this exercise, make a mental note of *which level of arousal you're experiencing.* Although you are likely to become aroused during the course of this exercise, orgasm is not the aim of the exercise. The aim of the exercise is to discover the wide range of response that exists between ice cold and orgasmic.

> **1.** Lie down on your back. Take a few deep breaths. Relax. Feel the air touching your skin. Feel your heart beating. Close your eyes.
> **What level are you at?**

2. Using your fingertips and starting at the very top of your head, slowly run your fingertips down either side of your head, keeping a light touch as your fingertips stroke the length of your hair. Enjoy all of the sensations that are created as you stroke your hair in this gentle fashion.
What level are you at?

3. Continue down your body. Begin stroking your neck and collarbone with the same gentle touch. Concentrate on feeling every nerve ending responding to the stimulation of your fingertips.
What level are you at?

4. From your collarbone, continue to your breasts and nipples. Go as slowly as you can. Feel the texture, temperature, and shape of your breasts and nipples. What is happening to your body?
 • Are your nipples becoming hard?
 • Is your rate of breathing changing?
 • Are you getting more aroused?
What level are you at?

Once you become acclimated to the stimulation and the intensity of the sensations begins to fade, continue down your body.

5. Stroke your sides and torso. Stroke your belly. Stroke your belly button. Ah, the belly button. A much overlooked, highly erogenous zone. Linger a little over that sexy, sunken little hole. Remember: keep it light and just use your fingertips.
What level are you at?

6. Now you're at the top of your pubic triangle. Lightly stroke your pubic hair. Slowly stroke the tops of your thighs and the sides of your buttocks. Focus on the sensations your touch is creating.
What level are you at?

7. Lightly stroke your pubic hair. What does it feel like to stroke yourself so close to your vagina without touching it? Is it exciting to you? Part your legs. Lightly stroke the clitoral hood. Stroke the entire vulva (your external genitalia). Stroke the outer lips, the inner lips, above, below, and around. Remember: You're not *trying* to stimulate yourself with this exercise, although you most likely *will* become stimulated. See how aroused you become *without* having an orgasm.
What level are you at?

8. Although it may be hard to tear yourself away from ground zero, continue down your body, lightly stroking the tops and sides of your thighs and buttocks. Stroke your knees. Slide your feet toward your butt so that you can reach and stroke your calves, the top of your feet, and your toes. Take your time and continue to use a feather-light, fingertip touch.
What level are you at?

You have just stroked your body from head to toe. How do you feel? What level *are* you at now? Do you feel:

- A sense of well-being? (Level 1)
- Warm and tingly? (Level 2)
- Hot and bothered? (Level 3)
- Explosively aroused? (Level 4)

You may have felt all of these various levels at different stages of the exercise. How does it feel to have completed the exercise? What is the lingering feeling?

Follow-Up to Exercise 1

Before your memory of the experience fades, look over the exercise again and take a minute to record your responses in your Bad Girl journal.

- What level of arousal were you at when you were stroking your head? Your neck? Your breasts?
- How long did it take at each station of your body before your arousal level started to climb?
- When is your arousal level the highest? When you first begin stroking your body, or after some time stroking your body? Is the answer different for different parts of your body?

Knowledge is power. When you are intimately familiar with your body's responsiveness to focused touch stimulation, you have the power to quickly increase your own level of arousal. You also have valuable information at your fingertips(!) which, when shared with your partner, will increase your level of pleasure, as well as provide a powerful new avenue of connection with him.

The Real "V" Word

Earlier in the book, I teased you a little when I referred to your voice as being the "V" word. I knew full well what your lusciously lascivious mind would think I was talking about! Well, I'm done teasing and now you really can go there; because I want to talk about it, think about it, look at it, name all of its parts, and get so comfortable and familiar with it, that you will never, ever think about it as an "it" again.

Are you a *Star Trek* fan? I hope so, because you're about to boldly go where you have never gone before. If you're like most of the savvy, "with it," sophisticated women it is my pleasure to work with either in my practice or in a classroom setting, your vagina is the Final Frontier of your personal anatomy. I sometimes refer to it as the dark continent, as it tends to remain as mysterious and unexplored as the interior of the African continent for far too many women. It's time for those dark days to end. I want you to become an expert on you, and I want you to become your biggest fan of your most private part, your vagina. Does that sound a little funny to you? It may sound funny, but if it does, take this little test:

Can you state the following sentences with a straight face and with conviction?

- "I'm *proud* of my vagina."
- "My vagina is gorgeous."
- "I love spreading my legs wide and displaying my vagina fully to my lover."

How'd you do? Are those statements true for you? Did you have trouble saying any of them? Did you have trouble saying all of them? When I reach this particular stage with a woman I'm seeing in a private session, I will sometimes ask her to read those very same sentences out loud to me. My God, the shades of pinks, reds, and purples she turns! The giggling! The hiding the mouth behind the hand! I sometimes feel as though I've stepped into a time machine and I'm a sex therapist in the nineteenth century! But it's the twenty-first century, and it's time for us to stop being ashamed of our vaginas.

Have you ever seen the movie *Fried Green Tomatoes*? Kathy Bates plays a woman who is going through menopause and struggling with all of the wild emotions that it's bringing up for her. She joins a "Womyn's Group," where she thinks they are all going to swap recipes and discuss the double coupons being offered at the supermarket. She goes to her first meeting and everyone is sitting in a circle on the floor of someone's house with a small mirror in front of them. The group leader instructs them to peel off their panties and look at their vaginas. There's this hysterical moment when Kathy Bates's face registers about fifteen different thoughts and feelings ranging from confusion, to nausea, to out and out fear.

It's funny in a movie, but it's not funny in real life. To me, it's sad that a woman in today's life and times could be so disconnected from the essence of her own womanhood. I don't want that to be you in ten, twenty, or thirty years; do you?

Besides, **men love vaginas.** *They get turned on looking at them.* They also get turned on by the way they feel, smell, and taste. That being the case, why do you work so hard to keep yours under wraps? It's time to look at your vagina in a whole new light (with lights *on* for starters, instead of *off*!)

Bad Girls Know Their Bodies

Finding the Erotic Artist Within

Have you ever taken a figure-drawing class? If you have, then you're aware that often times the models who pose don't have the body type that is held up as today's ideal. They're often quite zaftig and voluptuous by today's standards. The first time a live model of substantial proportions unveils herself in front of you, you may find yourself fighting off the urge to give a little giggle; it can take many minutes before your judgmental mind shuts off. But as you start to draw, you stop *looking* at your model and you begin *seeing* her. Every ridge, curve, and fold becomes fascinating and wonderful; your model becomes absolutely beautiful to you.

In this next exercise, you are going to be your own model. You are going to employ that same appreciative eye of the artist with the most intimate part of your own anatomy. It doesn't matter if you're a Rembrandt or if you struggle with stick figures; your level of artistry is not important. What *is* important is that you begin to see and relate to your vagina in a whole new way. Now don't forget: you're in figure-drawing class, so show some respect . . . and no giggling!

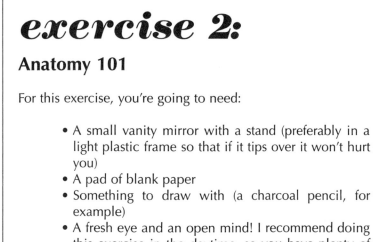

exercise 2:

Anatomy 101

For this exercise, you're going to need:

- A small vanity mirror with a stand (preferably in a light plastic frame so that if it tips over it won't hurt you)
- A pad of blank paper
- Something to draw with (a charcoal pencil, for example)
- A fresh eye and an open mind! I recommend doing this exercise in the daytime, so you have plenty of light to see the particulars.

1. Prop yourself up on your bed with lots of pillows behind you. Get nice and comfortable. You can be completely naked, or naked from the waist down.

2. Spread your legs until they form a "V." Draw your feet towards you until your feet are resting flat on the bed. Place your mirror at an angle that allows you to see your vagina clearly.

3. In order to get an unobstructed view, place your pad of paper on top of your knee or thigh. Your sketch is going to include your entire vulva, so begin your sketch at the top of your pubic triangle and work your way down to your *mons veneris*. Mons veneris is Latin for "hill of Venus" (Venus being the goddess of love, of course), and it refers to the pad of fatty tissue that covers the pubic bone. The pubic bone is below the abdomen, but above the labia. This little layer of fat protects the pubic bone from the impact of sexual intercourse. It is also a highly erogenous area for many women; you may have discovered that yourself during the sensate focus touch exercise.

4. The next part of your sketch should focus on the *labia majora*. The labia majora are the outer lips of the vulva. The word "lips" can be a little misleading, as often the labia majora are more like elongated pads of fatty tissue that are found on either side of the vulva. The labia majora are usually covered in pubic hair and contain numerous scent-producing glands. There is every reason to believe that these scents are a sexual stimulant.

5. Now it's time to draw the *labia minora*. The labia minora are the inner lips of the vulva. These "lips" are sometimes enveloped by the labia majora. If you don't see these lips, spread the labia majora apart with your fingers; the two thin stretches of

protruding skin that you see are the labia minora. These lips protect the vaginal opening. They can vary widely in size, shape, and appearance. Some women can't see these lips without pulling the outer lips aside; on others, the lips are always visible, as they are long enough to protrude beyond the outer lips. It is the labia minora that often inspire comparisons to parts of a flower (I think of orchids, personally), and both they and the labia majora are extremely sensitive to pressure and touch.

6. Time to draw the clitoris. Just so we're all on the same page, your clitoris is the small, highly sexually sensitive little button of pink or white flesh that is located just above the top of the labia minora, and under a retractable hood of skin. The technical term for the clitoral hood is the *prepuce*. When you are sexually aroused, your clitoris engorges with blood and can distend past the prepuce in order to facilitate manual stimulation. It is the same physical response that occurs in an uncircumcised male. Some women have a very small clitoris; and others have a clitoris that is large enough to extend past the prepuce even in a non-aroused state.

7. Spread your labia minora apart with your fingers and draw the opening to the urethra. The urethra is the small membrane-covered hole just below your clitoris. The urethra, or urinary tract, is connected to the bladder; the small hole you see is where you urinate from. Although located between two of your sex organs (your clitoris and your vagina), the urethra itself is not a sex organ; although try telling that to women who like their urethra gently stroked and licked! (Just an aside: because the urethra is in the same general neighborhood as the anus, always wipe starting from the urethral opening toward the anus, and not the other way around to avoid infection.)

8. Like the urethra, the vaginal opening is nestled between the lips of your labia minora. Your vaginal hole is directly beneath your urethra. The opening to the vagina can be anywhere from half an inch to two inches wide. Although you can't see them, directly on either side of your vagina are the Bartholin's glands. These glands produce a small amount of lubrication when you become sexually excited. What does your vaginal opening look like? Is it a small "O" shape? Is it a slit? An oval? Draw it now.

9. The final subject of your anatomical still life is the perineum; the short, smooth, stretch of skin that starts at the bottom of the vulva and extends to the anus. Although not technically a sex organ, it can be quite arousing when this area is stroked, licked, or caressed.

Your intimate portrait is now complete.

I hope that seeing yourself with the eye of an artist has helped you to feel more comfortable with yourself, more accepting of yourself, and more appreciative of your own inherent beauty. Besides learning the actual names of all your parts, the other aim of this exercise was to get you used to confidently displaying your beautiful vulva. Good Girls are exhorted from very early on to "keep your knees together." It can go against every grain and fiber in your body to keep your legs spread and display your vagina for an extended period of time. But you have to be able to spread your legs for yourself before you're going to be able to keep them spread for someone else. And there is *nothing* so exciting, sexy, or truly Bad to a man as a woman who is able to proudly present her vagina to him.

So no more hiding, shunning, or shaming it. It's a new day, it's a new you, and your new relationship with your vagina has begun.

You're Getting Warmer . . .

Now that you've gotten to first base with yourself(!), it's time to go even farther. You just performed a general, full-body sensate focus touch massage. Things are about to become a lot more specific!

In the next exercise, you're going to focus on the incredible sensitivity and amazing range of stimulation and arousal you can experience by deeply massaging the area *surrounding* your clitoris. There are only two rules: You're not allowed to touch your clitoris and absolutely, positively, *no orgasms*! The purpose of this exercise is to tease yourself to new heights of arousal, eroticism, and stimulation without direct contact. Let the games begin!

exercise 3:
The Clitoral Clock

For this exercise you might want to use some KY Jelly or another kind of sexual lubricant. It isn't a necessity in order to complete the exercise, but it might make it even more fun! Indulge yourself in some soft music, scented candles, and gentle lighting, too; you deserve it.

1. Lie back on a soft, comfortable surface. If you are using oil or jelly, place a towel underneath you. Allow yourself to relax completely. Take several conscious breaths. Focus on the exhalation.

2. Part your legs until they form a wide "V." Applying firm pressure and using just the pads of your two middle fingers, slide your fingers down your pubic hair until they are just slightly above your clitoris. This position is **12 o'clock** on your *clitoral clock*. Let your fingers rest there for a while. What level of arousal are you experiencing? No stimulation

(Level 1)? Some stimulation (Level 2)? Remember: *Do not touch your clitoris.* It's a no-no in this exercise.

3. Now slowly move your fingers in a clockwise direction until you come to 1 o'clock. Keep the pressure firm. Although you may be feeling kind of tingly, *do not touch your clitoris.* You can masturbate to orgasm *after* the exercise if you want to. Right now we want to excite your clitoris by coming close, but not *too* close. How does 1 o'clock feel to you? What Level are you at?

4. Continue slowly going around the face of the clock in this fashion, noting at 2, 3, 4, 5 o'clock, etc., what level of arousal you are experiencing. Go around the face of the clock several times. Try varying the speed and level of pressure that you use with your "sweep second hand."

This exercise can be extremely effective for women who struggle with low levels of arousal. Taking the attention and pressure off having an orgasm can work wonders. This is definitely an exercise to share with your partner, so that he can play "rock around the clock" with you!

Cruising the Love Canal

Now that you are on speaking terms with the exterior parts of your sexual organs, it's time to look within and discover some of the mysteries and miracles to be found inside the vaginal canal itself. We've come a long way since the pioneering sexual response researchers Masters and Johnson first told us in the 1960s that the *only* way a woman can experience orgasm is through direct stimulation of her clitoris. Although it was an important step in opening up the entire subject for discussion and exploration, the supposition was, nonetheless, incorrect. There are *many* ways that a woman can have an orgasm; not the least of which include nocturnal emissions—better known as a wet dream (yes, guys aren't the only lucky ones, women have them, too!). Don't get me wrong; I'm all for orgasms produced by direct clitoral stimulation! It's just that I want you to be aware of *all* of the different ways your body is designed to give you unlimited pleasure. And I want you to know how to access that pleasure, at your command.

G! That Feels Terrific!

You know the basics. You know how good it can feel when a man's penis is inside you. You may have even had a vaginal orgasm during intercourse a few times. But have you ever wondered why you don't *always* have an orgasm during intercourse? Why sometimes, but not others?

The answer may very well lie just beneath the surface and a few inches into your vagina, in that area known as the *G-Spot*. You've probably heard of the G-spot (the "G" stands for Grafenberg, the name of the gynecologist who first wrote about the spot's existence), but experience has shown me that most women think of the G-spot in the same way that they think of unicorns and the tooth fairy: a lovely but unsubstantiated myth. Well Virginia, there really is a Santa Claus, because the G-spot is as real as the nose on your face. Once you know where to find it and how to stimulate it, it will bring you a lot more pleasure than scratching your nose does! But talk is cheap, and it won't make a speck of difference in your life unless you can prove to yourself that what I'm saying is true.

exercise 4:

Here, Spot!

As always, privacy, comfort, and a pair of clean hands are needed to complete this exercise. In order to be able to relax into the sensation of stimulating your G-spot, be sure to urinate before you begin.

Please keep in mind that this exercise (as well as the many others in this book) is designed to give you pleasure. **If something doesn't feel good to you, or you are experiencing discomfort, by all means *stop*.** Stop *immediately* and call your doctor. Although there is nothing dangerous about inserting your finger into your vagina, you should always listen to your body and respect the messages it sends you.

1. Lie on your back. **Breathe deeply**, and *relax*. Insert your middle (longest) finger into your vagina (use care if you have long nails!). If this your first time ever exploring your vagina, you can feel that the walls are not smooth, but kind of corrugated—like fleshy cardboard. Sounds awful, yes, but the better to please you, my dear! Your G-spot is located on the upper (front) vaginal wall. In order to locate this area, crook your finger slightly toward yourself until you can feel the ridge of your pubic bone underneath the skin and muscle. Your G-spot, or G-"area" as the case may be, is beneath the surface of the skin; it is not located on the surface of the skin itself.

2. Gently rub the pad of your finger back and forth, or up and down, over this portion of the vaginal wall. Use enough pressure so that you are actually massaging the area beneath the surface skin. Note: Some women's fingers may not be long enough to reach this high in their vaginas. In that case, a small investment in a gooseneck dildo is highly recommended. You'll be glad you did!

3. The vaginal wall may feel a little rough at first, but with continued stimulation, the area will swell and begin to feel soft and pillowy. If several minutes elapse and you aren't experiencing any sensations of arousal, experiment with different areas of the vaginal wall. Your G-spot may be located either higher or lower along the wall. You can also try inserting a second finger in order to apply more pressure to the spot.

4. As you explore your vagina, you will probably encounter your cervix along the way. Your cervix feels like a hard knob at the top of your vaginal canal. Experiment with applying a little pressure to your cervix using your finger. Although some women experience a little mild cramping when they rub their cervix, for most it is a very good feeling.

Your cervix, and the area directly behind it, are known as the *X-spot* (for ecstasy, perhaps?) To access the area behind the cervix, bear down on your finger a little bit until you can feel it slide behind the knob of the cervix. Use a gentle massaging motion with your finger. Does X mark the spot for you?

5. Slide your finger back down to your G-spot area. Pay close attention to the levels of arousal you are experiencing. Does continued stimulation take you to a Level 2? To Level 3? To Level 4? Breathe, breathe, breathe.

6. It is through stimulation of the G-spot that some of our more fortunate sisters experience what is known as a *gusher*. A gusher is a type of orgasm wherein the woman literally ejaculates from her vagina or her urethra, just as a man does from his penis. The ejaculate itself (which is sometimes mistakenly thought to be urine), is a clear liquid, similar to a man's semen; but without the sperm, of course! Women who ejaculate report it to be an intensely pleasurable experience. Not all women ejaculate, and not all women who ejaculate do it every time they have an orgasm. There is a lot to be learned about female ejaculation; the world awaits your personal research!

Follow-Up to Exercise 4

Take a few minutes after completing the exercise to write in your journal. Among other things, you might want to ask yourself:

- How did it feel to explore your vagina to such an extent?
- Do you feel you know more about yourself than you did before the exercise?
- Were you able to find your G-spot?

- Did you become aroused by massaging your G-spot?
- Did you have an orgasm? If so, was it the same, more, or less intense than a clitoral orgasm?
- Did you ejaculate? If so, how did it feel?

Not to worry if you didn't find your G-spot, didn't become aroused by massaging the anterior wall of your vagina, or didn't have an orgasm of any kind. Many women can't reach their G-spots with their fingers and need a sexual toy or device that is specifically designed to do the job. Other women prefer to do the research with a real live penis, and they need their men to help them with the exploration. Later on in the book, you will find several sexual positions that are designed to make it easy for your partner's penis to stimulate your G-spot. If you weren't able to locate your G-spot during the exercise, *please don't give up!* It can take several attempts using different methods before you hit on the element or combination of elements that works.

Say Stranger, What's Your Name?

So far in this chapter, all of the exercises have focused on the physical aspects of knowing your body. But knowing your body takes place on a psychic and psychological level, too. The last exercise in this chapter is going to focus on strengthening the psychic connection that already exists between you and your female anatomy.

Even though we all know that a "rose by any other name would smell as sweet," the word "vagina" is, nonetheless, a little tough to cozy up to. The word "pussy," mentioned in the very beginning of this chapter, does work for a lot of women I know, but is a little intense for many others. I have purposely used the word vagina a lot in this chapter, because I think it's important that women don't flinch when they hear it. But we're past that point now, and when I began this chapter, I mentioned that I wanted you to get so intimate with your vagina that you don't think of it as an "it" anymore.

One of the best ways I know of to personalize something is to name it. You name everything important in your life that you care about, don't you? You name your dog, your cat, your goldfish; some of us name our cars and even our houseplants! When you're in a relationship, an endearment or nickname often completely replaces your lover's given name. In fact, you may only use his proper name when you're ticked off about something!

Well, if it's okay to name a houseplant, then it's more than okay to name your vagina. You've been spending lots of quality time with her these days, haven't you? Gotten to know her a lot better? Grown fond of her personality, smiled at some of her quirks, marveled at her dimples, curves, and clefts? I hope that your respect and appreciation for your vagina and all that she does for you has grown over the past twenty pages.

In the next exercise, you're going to formally acknowledge your new relationship with your body and with your vagina. This acknowledgment is going to include a formal naming ceremony of your Pleasure Temple (how's *that* for a euphemism for vagina?)

exercise 5:

Name That . . .

Create the proper ambience for yourself. Light candles or incense. Choose some of your favorite instrumental music to play in the background. Make a sacred space. It's very clear that you are not the average woman! You are a woman who is committed to personal growth, personal bests, and serious Bad Girlhood. Allow your surroundings to reflect your seriousness in this endeavor.

1. You can sit cross-legged on the floor, on a chair, or recline in bed. Pick a position that is most comfortable for you.

2. Close your eyes. Place your attention on your breath, as you breathe deeply and fully. Let all the little stresses and worries of the day fall away. This is *your* time. Take a moment to reflect on all of the hard work you have already put into your program to become a genuine Bad Girl. Allow yourself to feel proud of your accomplishments.

3. Clear your mind. Now, *silently ask that your vagina's name be revealed to you.* Put the question forth three times. Then quiet your mind again. You may hear nothing for several minutes, or you may hear a cacophony of different names. The name may suddenly pop into your head out of the silence, or it may just rise to the top out of all of the other names that are floating around in your head. Let the names that make you giggle pass by—this is a serious matter. No need to force anything; have faith that the right name will eventually become clear. It may take one minute or twenty—enjoy the process!

4. Once the name becomes clear to you, say it out loud three times. Give thanks for receiving the name and for the new bond that now exists.

How does it feel to know your vagina's true name? Doesn't it feel good? It's no longer the anonymous boarder at the end of the hall, or the no-fly zone, or the Bermuda Triangle. It's a *she*, and she has a name! I know it may have seemed silly at first, but addressing your vagina by her proper name is a very loving and respectful way to approach yourself. A word to the wise: You might want to keep the name to yourself. Keeping it secret keeps it special.

I'm a big believer in what's good for the goose is good for the gander. That is why in this chapter, you've learned new ways to touch, tease, and excite *yourself*. Ladies, it's time to turn the tables. In the next chapter, I'm going to share with you all of the different ways a Bad Girl goes out of her way to drive a man absolutely out of *his* mind with desire.

Chapter 7

Bad Girls Touch and Tease

*C*ynthia has been living with Kevin for almost seven years. Approximately once a week for the past seven years, Cynthia and Kevin have made love. When Cynthia wants to have sex with Kevin, she doesn't have a problem communicating her intentions, she just gets into bed without any clothes on and waits for him to notice. Sometimes Kevin notices right away; other times, if he's really preoccupied, it can more than a few minutes. But once he notices, he's always cooperative, and their lovemaking quickly begins. Cynthia is not unhappy with the sex she has with Kevin, she just wishes from time to time that it had more sizzle, that it had more tension, that it had more . . . *something*. Cynthia feels that her sex life is good. She just wishes it was a little more Bad.

Cynthia's problem is not a problem with desire, it is a problem with the art of seduction. **Bad Girls believe in serious seduction, and they know that seduction isn't just a man's job.** A woman who knows how to seduce a man is a woman in a position of power, and a position of power should be your favorite position, because it is foreplay for all of the others.

Seduction is a game of tension and excitement—a game that calls for touching and teasing. Seduction is not a waiting game (waiting for *him* to make all the moves), nor is it a "take me, I'm here" game (like Cynthia's signature move). Seduction is a pleasure game that takes time to build, where no one needs to play the innocent. It is a game where the brush of a hand or the crossing of a leg can make a man want you for days and days, and where something as simple as the sweetness of your breath can make him remember you forever.

Bad Girls know how to play this game and they love it every time they win. Bad Girls aren't afraid to show interest, but they always know just how much to show. They also know when the overture is complete, and it is time for the performance to begin. Bad Girls aren't afraid to make first contact, and they aren't afraid to reveal their desire. Yet something about the way a Bad Girl does this always makes a man feel he is under her spell.

In this chapter, I'm going to teach you what Bad Girls know about the rules of this "touch and tease" game, and these are rules you will follow forever. Whether you've been with someone for years and years, or you met him for the first time last night, you can't be afraid to leave your man waiting—at least for a little while. The power of seduction is the power to thrill; and the chase should always be thrilling.

Where There's Smoke, There's Always Fire

As much as I love sex (and I don't have to tell you how much I love sex, do I?), I enjoy what happens *before* sex almost as much. What happens in a Bad Girl's world *before* having sex? The delicious tension that exists between a man and a woman; the longing, the electricity, the anticipation. A Bad Girl can create this scenario with just about anyone, anytime she wants, because a Bad Girl is skillful at the art of seduction— she has refined teasing to an art form.

Seduction is nothing more and nothing less than this: **One person creating a context for sexual thought that is then shared between two people.** The most skillful teases are able to create this context without the recipient even being aware that it's being done. Did you catch that part? He doesn't know he is the victim of a seduction—he doesn't consciously know what is happening. He just feels drawn to the seductress. Does that make it a manipulation? Perhaps, but one with the very best intentions, because you're not just playing, you're playing for keeps. Besides, a skillful seductress never makes the object of her desire feel manipulated. She just makes him feel *wanted*. All he really knows is all that he needs to know: That suddenly he is on an *unspoken* sexual wavelength with you—one where the two of you are sharing the exquisite sense that anything between you is possible. If that sounds like an unfair manipulation, then I plead guilty as charged!

How Does *She Do It?*

How is it done? How does a Bad Girl create a shared context for sexual thought without looking clumsy, without feeling foolish, and without being caught?

- A Bad Girl creates a sense of invitation and anticipation through the use of enticing self-touch.
- A Bad Girl gives a man a guided tour of her best features by directing his attention to different parts of her body through a technique known as channel switching.
- A Bad Girl leaves a man longing for eye contact.
- A Bad Girl knows just where to touch a man, and just how long to touch him.

And it doesn't stop there. Because once the chase is over and a Bad Girl has *allowed* herself to be "caught" (ha!), she knows just what to do to prolong the delicious teasing—taking it to the bedroom (or the room of her choice!). Now, we're going to get to all of this by the time this chapter is through, but all in good time, my pretty, all in good time. First I need to establish a few things—rules of the game, so to speak.

The Good Girl's Guide to Bad Girl Sex

Teasing Tip #1:
Good Things Come to Those Who Wait

So much in our culture is done quickly. We eat quickly, we drive quickly, we walk and talk quickly. But seduction, otherwise known as the art of touching and teasing, *cannot* be rushed. You absolutely, positively *must* take yourself out of the "instant gratification" mindset if you want to be a successful tease. A tease takes her time. Like a majestic cobra that hypnotizes its prey with its mesmerizing markings and swaying movements, a Bad Girl in control knows that a man under her spell is going *nowhere*. And she is in absolutely no rush to hurry the process along. On the contrary, sudden movements can completely break the spell and ruin the mood. So the first thing you have to remember when you are teasing a man is this: **keep it slow; slow and deliberate.**

Teasing Tip #2:
Think Honey, Not Vinegar

It sometimes seems that women equate being Bad and seductive with being cold and aloof. Let me tell you, speaking from years of both professional and personal experience, nothing could be further from the truth. It is possible to be friendly and warm and still be sexy, mysterious, and alluring as hell. It takes a little more work, because you have to work on lowering some of those anger-driven knee-jerk reflexes. But this charmed combination is the one that is most appealing (and usually, irresistible) to men. Put up too much of a wall and men will either think you're insecure, or find you unapproachable. Either perception is a definite seduction killer. You don't want to turn yourself into a target for a one-time-only conquest. You want to be the woman he can't get out of his mind, no matter how many times you've been intimate. So the second thing to remember when you're being a tease is to drop that icy façade, if it's something you have cultivated. **Think warm; warm and in control of your thermostat.**

Bad Girls Touch and Tease

Teasing Tip #3:
Be a Responsible Bad Girl

Once you become a world-class seductress, it can be easy sometimes to forget your own seductive strength and accidentally turn your charms and attention in the direction of men you *should* be leaving alone. I'm talking about inappropriate men such as your friends' husbands and boyfriends, your male co-workers, or your employees. Don't do it. Like a black belt in karate, it's important to remain aware and respectful of your abilities at all times, and only unleash your considerable charms on *appropriate* recipients. Bad Girls always maintain healthy boundaries in both their personal and professional lives. **You have to exercise self-control.**

Okay. So much for the ground rules. It's time to learn some new moves!

Switching Channels

There are all sorts of channels: television channels, psychics who channel spirits from beyond, The English Channel. What kind of channels could I *possibly* be referring to in this book? When I speak of a channel, I am referring to **any part of your body with which you can communicate.** Your eyes are a channel, your mouth is a channel, your facial expressions, your voice, your body language; they're all channels.

You know how easy it is to relax on the sofa with the remote control and effortlessly switch from one channel to another? You can instantly choose a comedy, drama, or news program, depending on what you want to watch. Well, switching your own channels is kind of like that, except that instead of being the viewer, you're the TV, and *you're* controlling what shows up on your screen. Once you become adept at channel switching, you will be able to instantly direct his attention to your pouty, sexy mouth, or your ravishing eyes, or your lovely smile, at will. Or to the nape of your neck, your shoulders, your breasts, or your calves. As the two of you are talking, you will be giving him a guided tour of all your best features, and most importantly, getting him thinking about you in a very physical way.

Tuning in to Your Finest Channels

Directing his focus to certain aspects of your physical features is primarily a mental process. You are not encouraging him to touch you (not yet!); you are offering precious images of you that register in his mind. This is a subtle, yet very effective way of encouraging a man to relate to you on a more intimate level.

Your most important channel, the one we're going to talk about first, is *your eyes*. Your eyes truly are the window to your soul, and when a man looks at you we want him to see that your soul is on fire.

Right now I'd like you to position yourself in front of a well-lit mirror. It doesn't have to be a full-length mirror, since you are going to be focusing right now on your face. As you look at yourself in this mirror . . .

- *Affirm to yourself that your eyes are your most beautiful feature.* You may not actually believe this to be true right now. That's okay. Once I'm done with you, they *will* be your most beautiful feature and we don't need any makeup to make that happen. For now, you can pretend you have Elizabeth Taylor's violet beauties, if that helps you—tell yourself whatever you have to so that you can act as if it's true for you.

- *Hold your own gaze.* As you continue to hold your own gaze, imagine that people are constantly telling you how beautiful your eyes are; you are fully aware that they have a powerful effect—a mesmerizing effect—on anyone you look at.

- *Think of your eyes as blazing suns.* If your eyes had the strength and power of the sun, you wouldn't look directly at anyone for too long, would you? You'd give people a full-on blast now and then, and then to give them some relief from the pure radiance your eyes project, you'd look down now and then to make sure you didn't blind anyone! Practice this kind of eye control as you continue to look at yourself in the mirror.

Bad Girls Touch and Tease

Here's the funny thing. . . . When you start acting *as if* your eyes are so beautiful and sparkly and radiant that you feel you have to protect people from looking at them for too long, two things will happen. The first thing that will happen is that the whole world will start agreeing that you have beautiful eyes. The second thing that will happen is that men will start *living* to be looked at by you. Looking into your eyes will make him feel as though he's practically seeing you naked. So *practice* looking at yourself in the mirror while holding these beliefs about your eyes in mind. Bathe in your own radiance. Do it. Feel it. Live it.

Mouthing Off for Good Reason

Now let's turn to the second channel: *your mouth*. Look into your mirror again and take some time to study your mouth. What makes for a sexy mouth? Isn't it a mouth that always looks like it's begging to be kissed? (Think Angelina Jolie.) What do you do when someone's about to kiss you? Don't you part your lips slightly and purse them a little bit? When a Bad Girl wants to get noticed, she knows just how to make kissing her a top priority for any man. Here's how you can tease and torture on a regular basis by having the sexiest mouth on the block.

- **Tell yourself you have the most beautiful mouth and most kissable lips on the planet.** You simply *must* believe this. If you believe that your lips are gorgeous, you will present them in a way that supports your belief.

- **Always be prepared to kiss.** No more tight, thin lines; no compressed lips; no stingy mouths. A Bad Girl always looks like she's ready to pucker. It's not necessary to have collagen injections, or to have lips like Julia Roberts, in order to pull this off. Just remember this: keep your lips and your mouth *relaxed*. As you look at your mouth in the mirror now, is your mouth looking relaxed and kissable? How much tension do you hold in your mouth? Tension turns a beautiful mouth into an unpleasant mouthpiece. Let that tension drop.

- **The next time you use a facial scrub, don't ignore your lips.** The sloughing action will exfoliate any dead, flaky skin. It will also increase the circulation, which will plump your lips up a bit.

- **Keep your lips smooth and moist.** A pure Vitamin E stick or other non-petroleum-based lip balm will keep your mouth its most kissable. Thanks to the miracle of modern science, you can also buy lipsticks that temporarily "pump up the volume" of your lips. Remember, you are putting your lips in a constant state of readiness: always ready to be kissed.

- **Practice, practice, practice.** It's the only way to develop comfort with your very sexy mouth. Make your mirror your friend, not a place to go for criticism. Practice at home relaxing the muscles of your mouth, parting your lips, creating a sexy pout, until you feel comfortable enough to incorporate this very sexy tease into your repertoire.

Time for a Facial?

The third channel of non-verbal communication is facial expression. What you most need to remember about your facial expressions is this: **They reflect your innermost thoughts.** So you can be *saying*, "Sarah always throws the best parties; she's a terrific cook." But if you are *thinking*, "I'd like to show you some of *my* signature dishes in private and with the lights turned low. . . ," that underlying thought will express itself in your face. Understand that this also works the other way: If you are out for a romantic dinner, and in the process of *saying* to your hunk-du-jour, "I'd like to show you some of *my* signature dishes in private with the lights turned low. . . ," but you are thinking, "I wonder if I'll be home in time tonight to tape David Letterman. . . ," your very unsexy underlying thought will broadcast itself across your face. In acting circles, underlying thoughts are called "sub-text," and are used to add richness and dimension to the dialogue. If you are *thinking sexy thoughts*, *you will look sexy having them*, regardless of *what's* coming out of your mouth. *If you are not thinking sexy thoughts, you won't look very sexy*, no matter *what* special words are coming out of your mouth. Every good actor knows this; now you know it too.

Working the Big Three

Your eyes, your mouth, and your facial expressions are three powerful nonverbal channels that can speak volumes without uttering a word. Once *you* are tuned in to the sensuality of these three channels, you can start to work them more effectively to your advantage. Every encounter with the object of your desire is an opportunity to give him a little taste of each channel. Since it is not possible for you to give equal focus to all channels simultaneously, you will naturally be switching focus between the channels. All you need to remember is that your focus is his focus— as you switch your focus from channel to channel, he is following right along with you, guaranteeing that this man you are teasing isn't missing one sexy thing about you. His process is not a conscious one, but yours *is*. You are in the driver's seat here, so choose your channel, choose another, choose another, and watch *his* attention move in complete rhythm with yours.

When you are learning to ride a bicycle, your focus is constantly switching between the three crucial elements (channels) of balance, pedaling, and steering. It takes a while to get the hang of this and create a rhythm to your channel switching that makes bike riding look so effortless. Like learning to ride a bicycle, you may have to master your sensual seduction ride one step at a time, gaining more control over each individual channel (eyes, lips, expression) before you become adept at channel switching. That's where your practice mirror can really help. But once you have individual control, it will be easy to start practicing your switching maneuvers. Once you learn how to make the switch, it is something you will never forget!

So much for the three basic channels—the beginner's channels. Are you ready for some more advanced channels? Channels that are strictly for an adult audience? Then let's continue.

You Can Touch Me There

You've seen it a million times and probably not even realized what it was you were seeing. What am I referring to? *Self-touch.* Self-touch is the great seduction technique that works so subtly, it completely slips in under the radar. If you want to see a great example of self-touch in action, you don't have to look any further than our favorite muse, Marilyn Monroe, in the movie *The Seven Year Itch.* If you've never seen the film (and you *should* . . . every Bad Girl should), all you have to know is that the setting is New York City during a summer heat wave. Marilyn is the upstairs neighbor of a married man whose wife is out of town for the weekend. Marilyn and the neighbor run into each other in the hallway, and he invites her inside to cool off in front of his air conditioner. Next to the famous-round-the-world scene where Marilyn's white dress billows up around her waist on top of the subway grate, the second sexiest scene in the movie takes place in front of that air conditioner.

Because the cool air feels so good on her skin, Marilyn can't help but touch her throat, the nape of her neck, her collar bone, behind her ear. Tom Ewell, who plays the neighbor, temporarily loses his ability to speak as his eye follows each millimeter of skin Marilyn's fingertips touch. Why has he lost his power of speech? *Because he is imagining HIMSELF touching, kissing, and licking her where she is touching herself.*

Touching yourself in a personal way in front of a man plants the subliminal seed of touching you in his mind. It is also an invitation for *him* to touch you everywhere you are touching yourself. That is the essence of self-touch, and I can think of no better example on earth than that stunning scene in *The Seven Year Itch.* Think of how many more channels this adds to your remote control!

The key to this particular form of sensual teasing is making it look natural and uncalculated. If it looks like you're *trying* too hard, it's not going to work. Remember this: If you're having a conversation with the handsome hunk, *only touch yourself while he is talking.* If you use the self-touch technique while *you* are talking, it will make you seem too self-involved. If you are with other people, or across a crowded room at a social function, *easy does it;* a little goes a long way. You're not massaging yourself, molesting yourself, or exfoliating yourself. Just a light stroke here, a soft caress there. Get the picture? Good. Now let's leave the world of movies behind and look at a real-world scenario to see how self-touch can be effectively used in your daily life.

Self-Touch Scenario

You're at a party. You're having a lively and interesting conversation with a man you'd like very much to get to know better. You're glad you're wearing the silk blouse with the Juliet neckline; it makes it so much easier to:

- **slowly stroke your left collar bone three times with the ring finger of your right hand while looking into his eyes (channeling, channeling) as he's talking.** After you've stroked your collar bone three times, just let your hand rest there.

He's not just good-looking, he's funny, too. As you begin to laugh, you:

- **throw your head back slightly and place your fingertips at the base of your throat. Slowly, slowly, let your fingers slide down your throat until they are drifting down toward your cleavage. Stop just below your collar bone.** Let your fingers rest there. As long as he keeps talking, you can keep your hand there. But if *you* begin talking, **take your hand off of your chest.**

The ball's back in his court. He's telling you about a passion in his life, sailing. As you listen to him, imagining what it would be like to have sex on the open sea, you:

- **slowly and gently stroke your bottom lip with your index finger.** Look intently into his eyes while you're doing it, and don't forget to smile. You're lost in a reverie, remember? You're not *purposely* being devilishly delicious—you Bad Girl.

Oh, the power in these small gestures! If he wasn't a grown man, I'd almost feel sorry for him, because he doesn't stand a chance against you. He won't even know what hit him; but he'll love it when it does!

Although self-touch is most hypnotic in an intimate one-on-one setting, you can use it the very same way if you're not in just-a-breath-away close, face-to-face contact with your victim. If, for example, you're eyeballing each other from a distance in a crowded restaurant, or across a conference table, or across a long line of Stair Masters at the gym, or, as the song goes, across a crowded room, the power of your self-touch gestures will still come across. Once he notices, it won't matter how many people are in the room: all he will see is you. Again, it can't hurt to *practice* the self-touch technique in private before you whip it out in public. After all, you don't want to give a man whiplash. And developing your personal style at home, with some playful in-the-mirror practice sessions, will give you that extra confidence you need to pull it off in public with panache and style.

Bridging the Gap with a Three-Second Touch

Okay. Enough about touching *you*—at least for now. What about *him*? When can you touch *him*? Here's a sentence worth committing to memory: When you're in the process of teasing a man, it's *very* important to touch him once or twice during the course of your conversation. Not fifty times. Think of *three* as the absolute maximum. (No matter how long the conversation—if you're planning on talking for a while, make sure to save at least one for later). Touching *him* bridges the gap. It's just a touch, yes. But it suggests a future of very intimate contact.

When you initiate gentle, intimate physical contact, you are letting a man know, through your actions, that it's okay for him to touch you, too, in the same gentle fashion. You're opening the door. You're not dragging him inside that door and ripping his clothes off, but you are making it clear to him that the door is not hermetically sealed. You are offering him a bit of hope. And every Bad Girl will tell you that nothing is more seductive than a little bit of hope.

Note that this touch should never seem overtly sexual or remotely calculated. It should be spontaneous, genuine, and sincere.

Bad Girls Touch and Tease

When to Touch?

Here are some of the best times, in the course of a conversation, for you to touch a man:

- When he makes you laugh
- When he says something you agree with
- When he says something that surprises you
- When your conversation is coming to an end

Where to Touch?

When you are seducing a man with your touching and teasing, *where* you touch is as important as when you touch. Touch him in a way that is too familiar and he may get the impression that you're overbearing. Here are the places you should *never* touch a man during your initial conversation:

- On his neck or face
- On his chest
- On his leg

When you touch him, touch him here:

- On his arm (either his upper arm, or his forearm)
- On his hand

How to Touch?

Keep your touch light, using your fingertips. No grabbing, grasping, or hitting (hitting is juvenile, and not at all Bad).

The touch should last *no more* and *no less* than *three seconds*. Any longer and it could seem cloying; any less and it may appear to be accidental, not leaving enough of an impression. The three-second touch is the touch that seduces.

"I'll Have the Combo Platter . . ."

Using channel switching, self-touch, and the three-second touch during the course of conversation are tried and true Bad Girl ways of turning an ordinary conversation into an extraordinary encounter. At first, these various techniques may seem a little awkward because there's a lot to remember and a lot to do. What happens over time, however, is that they evolve into a perfectly natural way of expressing your interest in a man. If you are feeling any hesitation right now, that hesitation will disappear the very first time you see the response these techniques can elicit.

Women, take note: This is not just a great seduction tool for a first date or chance encounter. It works just as well, if not better, when you and your intended share a little history. Just because you're already in a relationship with Mr. Wonderful, don't think you can't completely seduce him using the exact same techniques. These techniques *always* work—they don't come with an expiration date. And they are a powerful way—an *ideal* way—to add serious heat to an existing relationship that has started to cool. These techniques make what is old new again. Try them, you'll see.

Okay. Speech over. Where to next? Where to next, when all of this great flirting and teasing lands you the guy, along with a few dozen roses at your doorstep? Or when all this great flirting and teasing reactivates interest and enthusiasm in the guy you've been dating for the past six months, living with for the past two years, or married to for the past decade (and, yes, there may still be some roses at your doorstep)? How do you *follow* that winning 1-2-3 seduction combination? Put another way, if seduction is nothing more and nothing less than one person creating a context of sexual thought that is then shared between two people, once it becomes appropriate to pull out all the stops, *what are some of the ways a Bad Girl keeps the seduction alive*? As you've probably guessed already, you've come to the right place to get that question answered, because I just happen to have a few suggestions.

140

Advanced Degree Teasing

When all of your exquisite teasing and seducing has been successful in breaking the ice and you've made the leap from mere acquaintances to intimate friends, an even greater array of teasing techniques and practices opens up for you. But before we delve into them, I think it's important that you stop for a moment and take a look at what your attitudes toward teasing are.

Teasing has suffered a bad rap over the years. When I was growing up, being called a "tease" was a serious charge. If a girl called you a tease, it meant you were a boyfriend-stealing tramp! If a boy called you tease, it meant that you had led him on, or had made sexual promises to him that you didn't deliver on. Well, times have changed. We're not in high school anymore and labels like "tramp" carry no sway over us any more. You're not going to hold out a promise for anything sexual that you aren't willing to deliver on . . . eventually. Are you going to be a "prick tease"? Yes—and a very good one. But far from being insincere, you're going to be a *serious* tease; one who uses the promise of sex as a means of creating longing, desire, and ultimately, delicious fulfillment. But first, another bedtime story . . .

Warning: Bad Girls Take Sex Seriously

Allison wants to have sex with her husband tonight, so she decides to set a romantic mood. She lights a candle in the bedroom to let her husband know that it's a special night. She puts on some of her favorite lovemaking music to make it doubly clear. Then she greets him with an enthusiastic kiss when he walks in the door. Allison leaves for a moment to slip into something totally provocative—an ultra-sheer teddy that she purchased just for this evening—but when she looks at herself in the mirror she immediately starts to question whether or not she can really pull this seduction off. When she walks into the bedroom to show off her new purchase she starts making jokes about her weight. Her husband, trying to keep the heated mood, says to Allison, "I want you." Allison responds, "I want you too," but she can't finish this sentence without starting to giggle.

Allison and her husband will still have sex tonight, but the real turn-on is gone. Why? Because Allison has a difficult time taking her seductive powers seriously. Instead of allowing herself to release into her genuine desire and her genuine power to entice her partner, she feels more like an actress playing a role and trying to stay in character. Allison's husband loves his wife, but her mixed messages leave him longing for the genuine article he knows Allison has locked up inside.

If you're going to be a world-class tease, you have to take sex seriously. Bad Girls don't try to play the role of seductress or vixen, they are the embodiment of these words. When they wear something sexy there are no apologies. When they ask for something sexy there is no backpedaling. And when they *do* something sexy there is no schoolgirl giggling. Sure, they can laugh and joke and have lots of fun in bed, but it comes out of a wicked playfulness, not out of nervousness.

As you read through the remaining teases presented in this chapter, I know that it is not always going to be easy for you to follow the guidelines and instructions. Some of this stuff is going to make you blush, some of this stuff is going to make you a bit weak in the knees, and some of it is going to make you giggle. I understand. But I also understand that the blushing and giggling phase is nothing more than that—a phase. And you can move through this awkward phase in your Bad Girl development very quickly if you practice your lines, your gestures, and your attitude in front of a mirror until those giggles are gone. After all, *you* are your toughest audience. Let the mirror be your challenge, and don't quit till you've won.

What Makes a Good Tease?

Although I like to think of teasing as sophisticated play for adults, there are a few guidelines to follow so that teasing remains exciting and enjoyable for everyone involved. I've already told you the golden rule: get the giggles out. Here are a few more things to always keep in mind until you have become a complete natural:

- *A good tease means what she says:* Make sure you don't say or promise things that you don't intend to do. Sure, it may sound sexy and feel dangerous, but if it isn't something you plan to follow through on, it will only lead to disappointment and frustration for your partner. Part of being an effective tease relies on the knowledge that you're really going to deliver. Otherwise it's just a big time waster; no tension, no intensity, no intimacy. Renege one too many times and you're going to have a resentful man on your hands, and rightfully so. Don't make promises you can't keep. A good tease keeps her word.

• *A good tease has a sense of humor:* Enjoy yourself. Teasing *is* serious business—and I don't want to sound like I'm contradicting myself—but teasing is also how adults play. It doesn't have to be *deadly* serious to be effective. Yes, giggles are out, because giggles are a product of your anxiety; but sexy humor is never out. Try not to focus so much on the execution of the tease that you become too rigid to allow for something spontaneous and unexpected to occur (like laughter, for example).

• *A good tease doesn't overdo it*: Avoid running the danger of too much of a good thing. Teasing should be thought of as an exotic spice that is used with constraint and premeditation; a little goes a long way. No need to cram all the great teases you're about to learn into one week or one afternoon—if you use one every once in a while, your special teases will become something your lover will learn to look forward to, and never tire of.

advanced teasing strategy #1:

The "See You Later" Teases

These hot little numbers are quick, to the point, and extremely effective. A "see you later" tease is delivered at the beginning of the day to get your lover's attention *real* quick, and give him something to think about for the rest of the day. It's a sneak preview of things to come, and much of its charm lies in its element of surprise, as well as its brevity.

As you are about to see, there are many ways for you to get your message of desire across, depending on your own personal style. Take a look at the list of very naughty "see you later" teases that follow and pick a few of your favorites. Or maybe this list will inspire you to make up a bunch of your own. Regardless of which one(s) you choose, when your tease is done, be sure to give him a little pat where it counts and say the magic words, "See you later."

The French Tickler

When you and your lover come together for a routine good-bye smooch before you head off in different directions for work (or for play), open your mouth and allow your tongue to find its way into his mouth. Instead of the routine quick goodbye kiss, kiss him deeply as you caress the back of his head. Let it last many seconds. As your kiss draws to a close, give his earlobe a love-bite; then give his butt a squeeze for good measure. Whisper in his ear, "See you later." He won't be lingering at the office tonight!

The Morning Handful

I like to creep up from behind when I use this tease. Do it when he's brushing his teeth, dressing in front of the mirror, or eating his toast at the kitchen counter. Wrap your arms around him and give his back a full frontal embrace. Cup his groin area in your hands. Start stroking and massaging until you start feeling a response. That's when you stop. "See you later." Then out the door you go.

The Peek-a-Boo

This is a tease that reminds him that there's a woman underneath that business suit. And if you have exhibitionist tendencies, you're going to love this one. Even if your lover is used to seeing you in various stages of undress as you prepare for the day, there's a big difference between sneaking a peek and being flashed. Flash him your breasts, flash him your bottom in a pair of hot French panties, or give him a full body flash. Tell him, "You can see more later." How about heading for the door in a trench coat, turning around and saying, "I feel as if I'm forgetting something. . . ," and then opening the coat to reveal that you're naked as a jaybird. "Oh, yes . . . clothes!" Wrap him up in your coat with you, give him a deep kiss, and tell him you'll "see him later." (But don't forget to get dressed!)

Give Me a Hand, Please

This is a very hot little tease. Take one of your lover's hands in both of yours. Kiss his palm. Run his hand over your face. Close your eyes and use his hand to feel your neck, your chest, your breasts, and your belly. If you're wearing a skirt, guide his hand up your thigh and rub your vagina through your underpants. If you're wearing slacks, rub his hand up and down over your crotch through the material. When you've finished using his hand to pleasure yourself, slip a few of his fingers into your mouth. Look into his eyes and say, "See you later."

The 15-Second Genital Kiss

Begin this tease by saying to your man, "Come here; I want to give you something." Wordlessly unbuckle his belt, unzip his pants, and then wrap your lips around his most sensitive appendage. Fifteen seconds should be long enough to start the blood flowing and elicit a few moans. **That's when you stop.** Tuck him back in, give him a frontal love pat, and tell him you'll "see him later."

What are the things your lover likes best in bed? What are the things he most likes to do to you? A wonderful appetizer to great sex is to give him just a little taste of one of his favorite things. Give him just enough to make him hungry for much, much more when you actually do see him later.

advanced teasing strategy #2:

The Midday Direct-Dial

These teases come as a bolt of lightning from the blue in the middle of any ordinary day. The midday direct-dial is basically an urgent communication that you deliver to your lover in the form of a private phone call (on a secure line only, please!). What are you urgently communicating? Your burning desire for him, of course. It's simple, it's free, and does it ever do the trick. Are you ready to create your own sexy surprises to catch your partner off balance in the middle of the day and leave him hungering for night to come? Then, consider some of my favorite midday messages:

1. "I'm calling to let you know that I'm not wearing any underwear today, and all I can think about is squeezing you between my naked thighs."

2. "I'll be waiting for you when you get home tonight. You'll know how to spot me: I'll be the one in your bed . . . with no panties on."

3. "I just got so turned on thinking about what you did to me last night, that I went into the bathroom and masturbated until I came. You have to give me more tonight. I have to have you."

4. "I have a problem I hope you can help me with. I have a desperate need to suck your _____. Can you help me out?"

You can be as graphic as comes naturally to you. Only you can know what will sound genuine coming out of your mouth. The key to a successful sexy phone call is in sounding authentic to the recipient. He has to *believe* you, so you have to be telling the truth. Entice your man with one of these midday direct-dial surprises and you will both enjoy a tremendous feeling of connection and excitement throughout the day. When day turns into night, you'll both be ready to fulfill your promises to each other.

advanced teasing strategy #3:

Taking the Gloves Off

The sun has set, all of your skillful teasing has worked its magic, and the moment you've been leading up to has arrived. You have your lover right where you want him: in your bed, wanting you. But you've both enjoyed your role as seductress so much, you'd like to continue along those lines just a little bit longer. What's a Bad Girl to do? Strip! That's right—a full on, no holds barred, old-fashioned striptease. If you've never done a striptease before, you may feel more confident about what you're doing if you try it first *before* you have an audience. Once again, you can use a mirror to help you get the giggles out. Otherwise, damn the torpedoes—full speed ahead!

Taking It Off—Taking It All Off

You'll want sexy, sexy music to strip to. Dim the lights, and light a bunch of great-smelling candles. Wardrobe is important, so wear something that makes you feel really sexy, but gives you a few items to take off, too. Personally, I'm partial to a man's dress shirt, a loosely knotted tie, a man's hat, a push-up bra, and a garter belt worn with a G-string, stockings, and high heels (my viewing audience seems to be partial to this, too).

Ask your man to sit back, relax, and enjoy. Let the beat of the music move you. The key word to keep in mind when you are stripping is *slowly*. Slowly sway your hips from side to side. You can close your eyes from time to time, but be sure to make eye contact frequently. Let him see the desire in your eyes. Think of your body as being a secret, and every inch of skin you expose is like telling just a little more of that secret to your lover. Take your time with every button, every snap, every zipper.

Touch yourself in a sensual way. *Slowly* trace the contours of your breasts, your torso, and your hips. Hold your arm out and run the back of your hand down the inside of your arm. Pause after each step: remove a bra strap from your shoulder; pause. Unsnap a garter; pause. Unhook your bra; pause. *Make him wait* to share your secrets; they will be all the more exciting to him if you do.

Throw every article of clothing you take off to your lover. Show him your back and give him sexy looks over your shoulder when you finally remove your bra and your panties. Continue to gyrate, undulate, and rock your hips; make Mae West proud. Remember to keep it slow and sexy. You can leave your pumps on to help keep *him* pumped, and when you've completely disrobed, walk slowly over to the bed, and join your man.

Once you break the ice with a full-on striptease, you will never take your clothes off the same way again because you will know how every piece of your clothing and every gesture has so much sexual power. Don't be surprised if you find yourself incorporating at lease one or two elements of the striptease every time you undress in front of your man. You might even find yourself doing a little stripping solo!

advanced teasing strategy #4:

Teasing at Close Range

Now that you're finally within his reach, your partner may fall on you like a starving man at a buffet. But you're not through being a world-class "prick tease" just yet. You want to intensify his desire for you even more. This kind of teasing calls for getting up close and personal. This kind of teasing calls for the laying on of hands: your hands, on his body. This kind of teasing calls for a very special massage.

Remember the exercise you did where you stroked yourself everywhere *except* your clitoris? Remember how hot it made you feel? You can do the same thing to your man. Envision a diagram of arrows, placed in a circle, with the tips all aiming toward *his* sexual center. That is the direction your massage is going to go: toward your lover's penis. Every move you make, every stroke you take, is going to be headed in that direction—focusing his attention, his energy, his blood flow, into his beautiful member. But what are you *not* going to do? You're *not* going to touch his penis! You're going to come oh-so-close to touching it, but you're not gonna touch it. Not yet.

By focusing your touch on the areas that surround his penis, you'll be directing the attention of every one of his nerve endings to the one thing that *isn't* being touched: namely, his aching, throbbing, swollen penis. Will he beg? Probably. Will he moan? Most assuredly. But you can handle it; because you're Bad.

Here's how it's done:

1. If your lover still has any clothes on, help him to undress now. Rub your hands together to warm them so that your touch has heat.

2. Think of the base of his throat as being 12 o'clock. Place both hands there, and begin one long, *slow* stroking motion down his torso that ends just above the base of his penis. Don't rush off once you reach his pubis; when your fingertips arrive just above his penis, take a moment to rest them there—let him know that *you* know exactly what you're doing.

3. Rub your hands together to warm them again. Now move one hand up to 11 o'clock and one hand up to 1 o'clock (slightly to the right and left of the base of his neck). Bring your hands in toward the penis with the same slow, continuous stroke. Stop again just before touching the penis.

4. Keeping in mind the diagram of the arrows I outlined above, keep moving your hands one hour further apart on both sides, then slowly bring them into the center, ending each sensual stroke just before touching your lover's penis. For instance, 9 and 3 o'clock should find your hands at your lover's sides, 5 and 7 o'clock will take you to the outside of each leg, and 6 o'clock will bring you right up the middle from his legs.

Never let it be said that you are a *heartless* tease; if your guy is being driven out of his mind by your touch, you have the option of providing him with some relief by directing your stroke *away* from his tortured member. Just imagine the arrows radiating away from the center of the circle—that is the direction in which your strokes must go in order to shift the energy away from his penis.

If you want to be *really* bad, once your guy has become erect, **mix up your strokes.** Give him one away stroke for every three toward strokes you perform. Using this technique, you can play with his erection and prolong his sexual agony for quite some time. Believe me, it's the kind of agony he has been praying for.

advanced teasing strategy #5:

The Hot Rod

You've teased and teased and teased and taunted. Now he's moaning and groaning, and begging for relief. What do you do? It's almost time to put him out of his misery, but you're going to do it in true Bad Girl style.

1. Using the massage technique you just learned (in Teasing Strategy #4), direct the energy and blood flow into your partner's groin, and bring him to the fullest height of his desire.

2. Take off your panties (if you haven't done so already). Now place one of your knees on either side of his body so that you are poised on top of him in a straddle position, supporting your weight with your own legs.

3. Take your lover's penis into your hand and slowly lower yourself until you are close enough to him that you can rub your vagina with the head of his penis. Think of his penis as your own personal tool, and use the head of the penis to stimulate your clitoris. No fair masturbating your partner *or* letting him enter you at this point—you're still having your way with him. Right now, his penis is for your personal pleasure, and your pleasure alone. He needs to wait his turn. Don't worry; you're not being cruel—your partner is going to love every minute of this. So take your time, and really let yourself go. If you have an orgasm, so much the better.

4. Once you have used your partner to your satisfaction, slowly, slowly, slowly lower yourself over your lover's penis and allow him to enter you. Don't be surprised if your lover has an immediate orgasm. After all, you have teased him to the brink of madness. Oh yes . . . don't be surprised if he's not the only one to have an immediate response! Every bit of teasing you have been responsible for has also been working its magic on you!

Bad Girls Touch and Tease

As you have most likely already discovered for yourself, teasing is an erotic double-edged sword; it always seems to arouse the teaser as much as it arouses the "teasee." And the very best teases are the ones that bring everyone to the brink of orgasm. Contrary to the bad (and I mean that literally this time!) reputation teasing has earned because of shoddy execution in the hands of amateurs, *artful* teasing is a statement of true desire of the highest order. Teasing takes time, forethought, and energy, and it is a statement to the recipient that you care enough to seduce, entice, and arouse him in imaginative and creative ways. It is another Bad Girl signature that elevates sex to an art form.

So what are you going to do the next time you get called a tease? Flash your sexiest Bad Girl smile and say clearly and without apology, "absolutely!"

Chapter 8

Bad Girls Love to Climax

Amanda makes love to her partner Alan at least twice a week, but she has an orgasm during lovemaking no more than once or twice a *month*. Sometimes she fakes her orgasm and then tries to forget about it. Sometimes she just tells Alan, "I'm fine . . . really," and then tries to forget about it. And sometimes she finishes the job herself, quietly masturbating once Alan has fallen asleep.

Amanda loves the feeling of being close to her partner and she wishes she could always have an orgasm with him. But it isn't that easy for her. Alan often struggles with the nuances of her arousal, and Amanda is always ready to sacrifice her pleasure when it gets too exhausting or too complicated.

Is this story a little too familiar? Trying hard to protect your partner's ego and trying not to be too sexually demanding, many of us Good Girls have told our partners on more than one occasion that having an orgasm isn't always that important. Some of us have said this so many times, we're starting to believe it! Try telling a man that *his* orgasm isn't important; watch the way *he* reacts.

Your orgasm *is* important. Big-time important. Every Bad Girl knows that. You were designed to climax. You *need* to climax. And you need to climax really hard. You owe it to yourself, but you also owe it to your man, because nothing turns a man on more than watching his woman in the throes of orgasm.

This chapter is devoted to your orgasm. We'll talk about breathing exercises that enhance your orgasm. We'll talk about positions that enhance your orgasm. We'll talk about muscles that enhance your orgasm. We'll talk about words that enhance your orgasm, and we'll talk about ways your man can enhance your orgasm, too.

You don't need to fake it, you just need to make it happen.

In Search Of . . .

The Big O. Climax. Coming. Tipping your hat to the Man in the Moon. Whatever you call it, the quest for a great orgasm has been an acceptable topic of discussion among modern women for the past thirty years. But where are we *really* in regard to having orgasms? How many of you are like Amanda, just kind of scraping by on infrequent, or less than explosive orgasms? Aren't you tired of it? Wouldn't you like to know that YOU have the power and control to *insure* that each and every time you make love, regardless of the skill of your lover, you absolutely, positively, *will* have a bone-rattling, mood-altering, "hairs on the back of your neck stand up" kind of climax?!

Of course you'd like to know that. Well, here's the good news: The future is *now*, because you *do* have the power, *right now*. Orgasms of this magnitude can be a consistent reality for you, time after time after time. Are you willing to devote a few minutes a day to learning some simple steps that will give you the control you need to experience this kind of pleasure? If you are, then you're only a few weeks away from having the kind of orgasms that most women only dream about. And now that you're *such* a Bad Girl, just dreaming about great sex isn't good enough for you any more, is it?

We're almost ready to get underway. But first, two very important questions: Do you believe you deserve to have powerful orgasms every single time you have sex? Do you really believe you're entitled to that kind of pleasure? It's crucial that you answer those two questions honestly, because if the answer for you is no, you *won't* make the effort to do the exercises that follow, and you *won't* have the consistently fabulous orgasms you're about to read about, because you don't believe you deserve them! It's so important that you know deep down inside you that you are worth this effort and that your sexual pleasure is simply not negotiable. The universe has given women so many different ways to have an orgasm, how could you think for even a minute that you deserve anything less than complete satisfaction? Can you say "yes!" to these questions? Can you say "YES!" so loud that it chills you to the bone? Good. Then read the following paragraph aloud and paste it in your Bad Girl journal so you can always find it, and always feel it.

> *From this point forward, I dedicate myself to accessing all the sexual pleasure my body is designed to give me. I now know that spine-tingling orgasms are my birthright, and I welcome and accept this pleasure into my life. I deserve supreme sexual pleasure and fulfillment. It is natural for me to experience this pleasure during every sexual encounter. I am willing to take the steps that will put me in greater control of my body, and that will allow me to experience the ultimate in sexual pleasure. I dedicate myself to enjoying all life has to offer, including incredible orgasms. I deserve nothing less. And so it is!*

If you have been following the road I've paved in this book, you have done a lot of work. Now that you are free of the last remaining remnants of the Good Girl mindset that have kept you from pursuing your complete, total, and absolute sexual satisfaction, it's time to fill up the space you've created with new information, techniques, and creative sexual ideas. Sound like fun? I thought it might. You're about to become a veritable expert at orgasm; both yours *and* his. It is a skill your man will treasure, your friends will envy, and one you will wonder how you ever lived without.

I'm Coming!

You know how a barbecue starts with the coals burning a little around the edges, and then the heat spreads to the other coals, and before you know it, the coals are so hot that anything that comes in contact with them immediately goes up in flames? That's the same guiding principle behind two sexual techniques called *peaking* and *plateauing*. Peaking and plateauing involve building a foundation of sexual arousal and desire to such an extent that you won't be able to help but fall over the edge into orgasm. Peaking and plateauing will also familiarize you even more with your own sexual wiring, giving you greater control over your sexual experience. There are two main components to the process of peaking and the process of plateauing: touch and breath. I will describe each piece clearly as we start the exercises. If you're groaning a little bit right now, and thinking, "Not more exercises!," remember this: Peaking and plateauing will increase the number of orgasms you have, enhance every orgasm you have, and, if you are a woman who has trouble reaching orgasm, break through any physiological barriers that have been holding you back.

All About Peaking

You may not realize it, but you have already practiced a truncated version of the peaking technique during the sensate focus touch exercise you performed earlier in this book. So this is going to be an easy one. During that previous exercise (see chapter 6), you gauged your level of arousal on a scale from 1 to 4: Level 1 being very little arousal and Level 4 being hot, hot, hot. *However*, during that exercise, even though you stroked yourself all over, you weren't trying to stimulate yourself directly. In fact, you were trying to avoid any intense stimulation. My. Oh my. Such restraint! What *was* I thinking?

Time to turn things upside down. In order to practice peaking, you're going to use the sensate focus touch *only* on your clitoris and vulva area. And instead of avoiding direct stimulation, you will very purposefully caress your genitals, learning to modulate your arousal so that it goes up and down in a series of peaks that are completely under your control. Why? Because having consistent, seriously mind-boggling orgasms requires having serious control over your sexual response. And the surest way I know of to gain this kind of control is learning how to attain and maintain whatever level of sexual arousal you choose. You have to be in charge here, moving your body through peaks and valleys as deftly as a fighter pilot maneuvers a jet.

Practicing peaking (and plateauing) may seem a bit complicated at first, as it asks you to approach your orgasm in a fairly unromantic, nonspontaneous manner. But within a very short time, the clinical quality of it completely goes away. Before long, all you know is that you are coming harder, longer, and more often than ever before.

It is really helpful to be in a relaxed, stress-free mood before you attempt the peaking exercise. So have a nice meal beforehand. Treat yourself to a leisurely bath. Set aside at least an hour for yourself and create a sensuous, warm environment with candlelight and soft music. Make it a fun adventure, not homework!

exercise 1:

A Peak Experience

The scale that is used for peaking and plateauing is from 1 to 10.

- 1 equals no arousal
- 2–3 equals a twinge of arousal
- 3–4 equals a steady, low level of arousal
- 5–6 equals a medium level of arousal (light lubrication)
- 7–8 equals high level of arousal (increased heart rate, intense breathing)
- 9 equals the brink of orgasm
- 10 equals orgasm

Follow these steps:

1. Breathe deeply through your nose and exhale slowly through your mouth. Feel yourself relax more deeply with each subsequent breath. Take several minutes to let the breaths relax and revitalize you.

2. **Begin to stroke your genitals in a sensate focus caress.** Re-acquaint yourself with the textures and shapes of the inner and outer lips, the clitoral hood, and the vaginal opening. Remember, the goal of a sensate focus caress is not to arouse, but to explore and experience. Arousal is often a byproduct of the sensate focus caress, but it is not your aim—*not quite yet.* My grandmother used to say, "You can't cook with cold grease!" Giving yourself a sensate focus caress insures that your "grease" will have plenty of heat when the time comes.

3. When you are at either Level 2 or Level 3 (twinges) on the arousal scale, **begin to masturbate with the express aim of raising your arousal level to a 3 or 4.** There is absolutely no need to put any pressure on yourself, or to feel any anxiety. No one is keeping a time-clock on you, and you are competing with no one. However quickly or slowly it takes for you to get there, is how long it takes for you to get there. It's all good!

4. When you feel yourself peak at the 3–4 level (a steady, low level of arousal), **stop stroking.** Breathe normally and allow your level of arousal to drop back down to level 1.

5. Begin stimulating yourself again. Let yourself *peak at Level 5* (feeling light lubrication). Stop stimulating yourself, breathe normally, and let your arousal level drop down to *Level 3*. See if you can make each cycle of peaking and dropping back down the scale last about five minutes.

6. Continue peaking up the scale until you reach *Level 9* (brink of orgasm). When you feel yourself going over the top, **begin breathing rapidly** as you *continue* to stimulate yourself with your hand and stroke yourself to *Level 10*. Bon voyage!

Don't kill yourself trying to peak up to Level 10 the first time if it's too exhausting. It is much better to spend as much time as you need to master peaking at the lower levels first, and *then* add the higher levels, than to build a wobbly tower on top of a shaky foundation. Don't push, don't force, don't rush yourself. Getting there is half the fun.

All About Plateauing

Once you master the concept of peaking and are able to bring yourself up and down the arousal scale, then you are ready to add plateauing to your sexual response repertoire. Plateauing is similar to peaking, but instead of hitting the peak and then sliding back down, you can hover a while at the top of the peak. This hovering, which typically lasts anywhere from ten to thirty seconds, creates a *plateau*. There is another difference between the two techniques: Peaking is achieved using manual stimulation (your fingers or other physical object), but plateauing is most easily achieved using your *breath*. I told you very early on that Bad Girls even breathe sexy; plateauing is the sexiest breath of them all.

exercise 2:

Plateau for Pleasure

Prepare as you did for the peaking exercise. Have a nice meal, a warm bath, and create the proper mood for yourself. Don't forget what my wise, old grandmother said!

1. Start with—you guessed it—a sensuous, genital self-caress. Breathe deeply. Feel your body relax more fully with each breath.

2. Begin the peaking process. Manually stimulate yourself until you reach Level 4 on the arousal scale. Try to remain at Level 4 for thirty seconds or so using your hand.

3. After thirty seconds, **remove your hand and take two deep, slow belly breaths.** This will make your arousal level drop down more quickly to a lower level.

4. When you feel you have reached Level 3 on the arousal scale, **begin *panting*—breathing very quickly**

in and out through your mouth—until you are back at Level 4 on the arousal scale. Experiment with going back and forth between Level 3 and Level 4, just by increasing or decreasing the speed of your breath. *If, however, you feel yourself becoming light-headed, stop panting.* Your body may have to get used to you taking in so much oxygen on a slower, incremental basis. Otherwise, continue peaking at slightly higher levels, and plateauing at those levels using the panting breath.

5. When you reach Level 9 and you are very close to orgasm, **cease all physical stimulation of your body and *pant* yourself over into climax.**

Did you get there on the first try? If not, give yourself a day's rest and then try again. You can do it. Maybe not right away, but very, very soon.

Can you see how dynamic and helpful it could be to use these peaking and plateauing techniques when you are making love? Can you see how peaking and plateauing can keep you orgasm-focused, even if your lover loses his focus (or has no focus)? Can you also see how training yourself to use your own breath to help you achieve intense levels of arousal makes it far more likely that you can tip the scales into orgasm even when the physical stimulation isn't enough to do so?

If you reach a plateau in your plateauing (i.e., you can't get to the higher levels of arousal), don't get frustrated. Just continue to practice the exercise. The key to getting past the stuck places is in not giving up. Besides, the more you do this exercise, the more you will grow to love it. It's exhilarating to see the control you have over your own sexual response grow more consistent, more precise, and more adept.

You may have been a knitter, a sewer, or a flute player in your former life, but now you have a new hobby: orgasmologist! Peaking and plateauing are the fundamental skills that are necessary for achieving Bad Girl type orgasms on a regular basis. The more time you spend practicing the peaking and plateauing techniques, the more quickly you will gain the control you need to reach dazzling new heights in orgasmic pleasure.

Bad Girls Love to Climax

Getting Your Breasts "Done"

You're about to be *so* happy I taught you how to peak and plateau! Now I'm going to teach you how to use those techniques to create another, very different, equally thrilling kind of orgasm. I'm talking about breast orgasms. And no, your eyes don't need to be checked—I actually said *breast orgasms*. It's not completely off the wall. Think about it: If you can have an orgasm in your sleep without even touching yourself, why wouldn't you be able to have an orgasm by stimulating your sensitive breasts?

Breast orgasms feel indescribably good. It's one of life's little ironies that such a fantastic orgasm can be achieved without even touching your vagina, but it's absolutely true, and you're about to find out for yourself. We'll start with a bridge exercise that introduces your breasts into the orgasm equation, and then we'll follow with a breasts-only orgasm exercise that will leave you breathless and braless!

exercise 3:
Global Warming

As you know by now, all good things begin with a sensate focus genital massage. Don't rush, and don't cut corners. Give yourself the same attention you would want your lover to give to you. Be fully present.

1. Once you are relaxed and breathing deeply, begin the peaking and plateauing sequence.

2. Bring yourself up to arousal Level 3 and maintain there for half a minute. Then stop stroking, and take two deep breaths to help you drop down to a 1 or 2. Then pant your way (plateau) back up to Level 3 or slightly above. Increase your arousal, level by level, breath by breath. No need to rush. Take your time and enjoy the process.

3. When you feel yourself reaching Level 9 on your arousal scale, **use one hand to continue masturbating, and the other to stimulate and massage one of your breasts.** Give the nipple special attention. Along with this physical stimulation, use the panting breath to keep your arousal levels high.

I dare you not to come.

exercise 4:

Global Meltdown

After you've accomplished Global Warming several times, you can move on to the Global Meltdown. Everything is the same as in the previous exercise, except:

1. When you hit peak Level 9, and you are on the brink of having an orgasm, begin the panting breath plateauing technique and **move *both* hands to your breasts.**

2. Give your PC muscle (that you've been strengthening every morning) a few good squeezes, and massage your breasts and nipples as you peak over Level 10 into orgasm.

Keep practicing, and soon you will be able to reach orgasm *simply* from massaging your breasts. How BAD is that?

Orgasm Enhancement

So far in this chapter, the exercises I've introduced to you have required you to master specific, rather complex techniques. These techniques will guarantee you great orgasms for the rest of your life, but it's been a lot of work. That's why I also want to give you a few fast and easy ways that you can coax your body into climaxing—simple techniques that you can try *tonight*. I'm betting that the words "fast and easy" sound pretty good to you right now.

exercise 5:

The Clincher

This three-step technique is good for either enhancing an orgasm or encouraging a stalled orgasm to come in for a landing.

1. As you near orgasm, **speed up your breathing** until you are panting (sound familiar?).

2. **Vocalize.** Let yourself moan and groan out loud. If you are having dirty thoughts, speak them. Don't hold back—let go! Men love it when women lose themselves to such an extent that they're "talking crazy," and saying all sorts of filthy things. Free your speech and your climax will follow.

3. **Move your body.** Writhe around on the bed. Make really sexy faces. Lift your pelvis off the bed and move your hips and torso from side to side. *Clinch* and then *relax* the muscles in your arms, your legs, and your toes. **Begin pulsing your PC muscle every few seconds. Continue clinching your PC muscle as you go over into orgasm.**

The Clincher incorporates a tai chi principle that is based on using the energy (positive *or* negative) that comes toward you. This is a great exercise for women who experience anxiety as they approach orgasm because it can actually help you harness that anxiety (anxiety *is* energy) and make it work *for* you.

exercise 6:

PC Passion

Don't be confused; this next exercise has absolutely nothing to do with being politically correct! It's another simple technique that intensifies an orgasm that is already heading your way using that beautiful PC muscle you've been working out like a pro. You have been doing your daily squeezes, haven't you? This simple technique turns your average orgasm into an "orgasm to the second power."

Here's the technique:

1. Use a sensate focus genital caress or the peaking and plateauing technique to bring yourself to a Level 8 state of arousal.

2. When you reach Level 8, insert your finger into your vagina. If you're with a partner, his finger will work just as well!

3. Practice tightening and then relaxing (pulsing) your PC muscle around the finger. Continue stimulating your clitoris and/or using your breath to maintain your arousal level.

4. This orgasm-enhancing technique relies on the *first strike* theory: **As you feel your orgasm approaching, intercept it with a first strike PC squeeze.** *Squeeze the PC muscle as hard as you can* before that first spasm of orgasm hits, and prepare for a mighty awakening.

You're going to love the way it feels!

Bad Girls Love to Climax

Your First "Air-gasm"?

We've all had it happen. You're enjoying great sex with your guy, but because of the way your body is positioned, a lot of air is getting pumped into your vaginal canal. Suddenly, your vagina is "whistling Dixie," or some other equally embarrassing tune, as the air makes it exit from the premises. Well, hold the phone! What if I told you that those little air pockets, or "vaginal turbulence," as I like to call it, could actually be a *good* thing? Well, it can be. The next time it happens to you, you can honestly say, "I *meant* to do that!

Your vaginal muscles and walls are constantly moving and changing position during intercourse. That's why air that enters your vagina while you're having sex can get trapped in air pockets inside the vaginal canal. This isn't happening because you had lunch at McDonald's. It's all completely natural.

Think of your vaginal canal as an inflated balloon for a minute. When you want to deflate a balloon, you can either untie the bottom of the balloon and let the air escape of its own accord, *or* you can apply pressure to the balloon and expel the air in one big gust. By applying pressure to your vaginal canal at the right moment, you can often *create* this explosive expulsion of air and this can *trigger* an intense vaginal orgasm. Do you want to see what I mean? Then try this next exercise.

---

exercise 7:
"I Meant to Do That"

This exercise is fun to try when you are already at a very high level of arousal, so wait till you're feeling mighty hot from some serious stimulation, then follow these steps:

1. The best way to encourage air to enter your vagina is by assuming the "doggie" position, so on your hands and knees you go. Bend your elbows and lower your upper body and head onto the bed.

Relax your back (if you can do so comfortably) so that you have a swayback. Your body should look like a droopy slant-board, with your butt being the highest point. Part your knees. You may feel a rush of air enter your vagina at this point. If that doesn't happen, pulse your PC muscle and imagine your vagina is swallowing air. You can do it!

2. When you can feel the air inside you, **straighten your back** while simultaneously tightening your lower abdominal muscles. Picture your vagina literally blowing the air out.

3. If you don't have a quick expulsion of air this way, try turning over onto your back, bending your knees and sliding your feet toward yourself so that you can hold your ankles, and pulsing your pelvis up and down into the air a couple of inches. Squeeze that PC. Maintain the image of your vagina blowing the air out.

If you often experience air entering your vagina when you make love, you can simply wait for the next time it happens and then try expelling the air on purpose. This is not pie in the sky stuff here, ladies. You've heard of women who can shoot ping pong balls across the room with their vaginas, haven't you? Well, how do you think they got their start?

Okay . . . It's His Turn

Enough about you. I've given you enough Bad Girl orgasm techniques to keep you coming well into the next century (and I've even saved a few more techniques for later). Time to turn your attention toward someone else who might also have an interest in a little sexual ecstasy . . . that's right, him! Your lover. Your partner. Your guy. Doesn't *he* deserve an evening, a weekend, or a lifetime of fabulous orgasms too? Granted, it's great to know that you can take care of business when you're the only one in the room. But when that isn't the case—when you've got some sexy company you want to play with—a Bad Girl's body of knowledge (or knowledge of the body, as the case may be) extends to the lucky man within her grasp.

Please Allow Me to Introduce Myself . . .

If penises could talk (can you imagine?), women wouldn't ever have to wonder about what feels good to the penis, how long to stroke it, or how hard they can squeeze. But penises don't talk, and often times, neither do the guys they're attached to! So a cycle of silence and ignorance often gets perpetuated, with women just kind of fumbling around down there, or simply avoiding the general area as much as possible.

Silence, ignorance, fumbling, and avoidance do not belong in bed with a Bad Girl. A Bad Girl takes as much interest in the penis as she does in her own vagina. Why? Because she *likes* it. In fact, she *loves* it. It's interesting to her, beautiful and exciting. Because she loves her partner's penis, she makes it her business to learn as much as she possibly can about it.

It always amazes me when I encounter a lack of curiosity in heterosexual women toward the penis. I have found that women often relate to their man's penis in the same way they relate to their automobiles: As long as they can hop in and get to where they're going, they're happy. They rarely lift the hood, read the manual, or check fluid levels. The only time they ever give it a second thought is if something goes wrong and it stops performing for them.

Not good enough. Not any more. *A Bad Girl is a penis specialist*. She knows more than the average woman—lots more. She never gets tired of playing with the penis, she never gets tired of learning about the penis; and she never gets tired of adding to her repertoire of penis-pleasing moves. So go grab your guy, tell him you're in need of some serious adult education classes that you just don't find at *The Learning Annex*, and get ready to know a good friend even better.

Jane, Meet Dick

Before embarking on an exploration of your lover's penis, it is essential that you approach the activity with the same respect, the same attention, the same patience, and the same sense of acceptance that you extended toward yourself when you were exploring your own anatomy.

It is essential that you refrain from saying or doing anything that could in any way shame, embarrass, or belittle your man in regard to his most private parts. Say the wrong thing and you may find that your first research expedition will be your last—and that would be tragic! So approach his penis with the admiration and affection it deserves, and you will have lifelong research privileges, I assure you.

exercise 8:

Slow Hand

Let your partner know ahead of time that the express purpose of this session is for you to become even more intimately familiar with his penis. Make sure he has nothing else pressing on his schedule because this might take a while! Why not start off with a warm bath together? Afterward, light a few candles, put on some soft music, and get busy.

1. Prop up some pillows so that your partner can rest comfortably in a semi-upright position. You will want to be able to gauge his responses to what you are doing, so make sure that you can easily see his face.

2. Start by giving his penis the same sensate focus massage you give yourself. **You aren't trying to intentionally stimulate the penis,** although that may of course occur. The purpose of this sensate focus caress is to become sensitive to the nuances in texture, temperature, and responses of your man's genitals; including his penis, the pubic mound, and the scrotum.

3. Use your fingertips, the back of your hand (be careful if you're wearing rings; you may want to remove them first), your open palm, and the flat surfaces of your fingers to very slowly touch and caress. Gently cup the scrotum and give a soft squeeze. Feel the way the testicles move inside the sac. Use your index finger to pet the head of the penis; run your

finger underneath its rim—the highly sensitive area where the head of the penis meets the shaft. Check the speed at which you're exploring and **slow it down by half.** Pretend that there's going to be a test at the end of this exercise, and you will asked to describe in detail every millimeter of his glorious genitalia. You want an "A," don't you? Take your time.

4. Is he getting hard? If he is, it's an indication that a soft, slow, gentle touch (as opposed to indelicately just "jacking him off") is an equally effective way to arouse him. What makes him moan the most? What seems to leave him cold? *Listen* and learn as you *touch* and learn. If he isn't showing any visible signs of arousal, *ask him* how it feels. *Just because he isn't getting hard, it doesn't mean he isn't enjoying every single moment.* If he *tells* you he isn't particularly enjoying it, that's okay too. Because this exercise is about you getting more tuned in to the sensitivity, vulnerability, and complexity of his penis. You're here to learn.

The Zen Hand Job

Have you ever watched a man masturbate? If you haven't, it probably won't surprise you to hear that men tend to go at themselves with the workman-like attitude of getting the job done quickly, and with as little muss and fuss as possible. They don't tend to linger at it. When a man masturbates, he just wants to hurry up and come so that he can put the magazine away, or turn the video off, or get out of the shower and get on with the rest of his life.

That's why when *you* masturbate a man, you need to be different. He already knows how to make himself come quickly, but what he *doesn't* do is make love to himself. And that's where you come in. As a certified Bad Girl, it is your aim, goal, and joy in life to keep your man's arousal level as high as possible, for as long as possible. When *he* masturbates himself, the memory of the orgasm fades as quickly as a sneeze, but when *you* do it Bad Girl style, he won't soon forget it. He'll be re-running the scene in his head on a continuous loop, and he'll get shivers every time.

Note: You need to get used to working with *both* hands. Most women use just one hand when they are handling a penis, but using both hands gets you fully *involved*. And that gets *him* fully involved—involved and excited! It also doubles the pleasure.

You can segue directly into our next exercise from the sensate focus caress in Exercise 8, or pick up here at another time. Whatever you do, get your guy to slow down before you begin! Get him to take a hot shower or bath beforehand. Don't just turn off the TV fifteen minutes before bedtime and hurry your way through this. Make it the main event of your evening activities. Also, check in with yourself to make sure you are up for it, and that you are in the right state of mind to devote your full attention, energy, and enthusiasm to the task at hand!

exercise 9:
Slippery When Wet

For this exercise, you will need a lubricant that is *specifically* designed by the manufacturer for use in a sexual context. Cooking oils, massage oils, baby oil, or any other type of oil or lubricant that is *not* specifically intended to be used on the genitals could cause extreme discomfort to your lover, or worse. If you don't already have a sexual lubricant on hand, you can skip ahead a little bit to the next chapter for information on what to buy and where to buy it.

1. You want to start with the lubricant preferably before your partner has a full erection. If he shows up for this exercise already fully erect, that's okay too—you can't keep some good men down. Pour a dollop of lubricant the size of a fifty-cent piece into the palm of your hand. Use the fingers of your other hand to spread the lubricant luxuriantly over the entire shaft of his penis. Use *finesse*. And don't be

afraid to use additional lubricant if you're not getting ultra-smooth contact. You're not rubbing hand lotion into the skin here, you are sensuously applying "sex sauce" to his penis, and it feels slick and wonderful to him.

2. Is he all lubed up? Good. Because I'm about to tell you the most important secret to giving an award-winning Bad Girl Hand Job. Listen closely: **When you give a man a hand job, don't think about touching him in a way that will make his penis feel good; think about touching his penis in a way that makes your *hands* feel good.**

Whenever I give that instruction, it always makes me feel like a Zen Buddhist or a Jedi Master. I know it seems like a minor distinction, but if you are able to make the switch in your brain, you will become a world-class penis manipulator, and your lover will consider insuring your precious hands with Lloyd's of London. (Of course, he'd be insuring the wrong part of you—it's your brain that is creating the magic.) When you are able to perform a hand job with this mindset, you instantly set aside all of your anxiety regarding: Am I doing it right? Does this feel good to him? Is this too hard? Is this too soft? The only person you are trying to please is *you*! So if the touch feels too light to you, it's too light. If it feels too fast to you, it's too fast. Simple, right? The best things in life usually are.

3. Try running one or two fingers up and down the length of the penis. Using the middle three fingers on both hands (using *both* hands is also a master stroke), gently press at the base of the penis, moving your hands around the circle like the face of a clock. Do try to avoid what I call "the angel's touch"—a touch so delicate that it barely registers on the "penis meter." Remember, his grip is probably a lot stronger than yours, and his penis has managed to survived a lifetime of self-gripping!

(I must note here that I love watching the penis as it begins to stiffen from the touch of my hand. It always reminds me of a sleeping giant that has been roused and is slowly coming awake. It never ceases to thrill me.)

4. Moving on. As his penis continues to harden, try alternating strokes using either hand. Go *really* slowly. Go back to pressing (more firmly this time) around the base of the penis every now and then, too. Keep his penis nice and wet—slippery wet—with plenty of lubricant. Don't skimp on the lubricant!

5. Experiment with different angles. Most women tend to hold the penis so that it is making a ninety-degree angle from his body (straight out). But you may discover that angling the penis up a bit as it starts to get hard—toward his stomach instead of straight out— keeps him a little more firm. A penis that is angled down—toward a man's legs—has the greatest tendency to lose its firmness.

6. Slowly, imperceptibly, begin a series of increasingly tight squeezes to the shaft of the penis. Squeeze, and back off. Squeeze a little tighter, and back off. Squeeze even tighter, and back off. Mix up these squeezes with slow but firm strokes, caresses, and finger rubs. (Remember: Whatever feels best to you!) Continue until he has an erection that looks like it's going to explode. Then, stand back! Because it very well might!

If pleasing *yourself* is the number-one secret to stellar manual manipulation, the number-two secret is to keep it *really slow*. That isn't to say that you should *never* move your hand quickly, but if you can make pleasing yourself and moving slowly the foundation of the activity, you will both experience a level of pleasure during the act that will be thrilling beyond measure.

Don't Talk with Your Mouth Full

No, I haven't suddenly morphed into Ms. Manners. I'm talking about more SEX, baby! Fabulous, wonderful, *oral sex*. I *love* to give head. Do you? If not, why not? Is it a confidence issue? Do you feel you don't know what to do? Are you afraid you're going to gag? Does that gorgeous monster scare you? That's not going to be a problem for long. Once you've finished with this exercise, you'll be able to charge for lessons.

Before we get down to the nitty-gritty, let's talk for a minute about the physiology of the male sexual response. A Bad Girl knows that no matter how hot she is, there are some men who just aren't quick starters. Some sleeping giants need more time to wake up and start to look like an erection. A Bad Girl is woman enough not to take that personally. She knows that some creative teasing and a little patience is all she really needs to pick up the pace. A Bad Girl also realizes that it's no reflection on her if a guy has a hair trigger. Some pumps don't need a lot of priming. The beauty of knowing the subtleties of oral sex technique is that one size doesn't have to fit all, and you can vary your methods to meet the particular need at hand. The possibilities are limitless.

> *BUT FIRST, WE MUST PAUSE. It goes without saying that if you are not in a committed relationship with a man whose sexual history and current health status you are intimately familiar with, YOU DO NOT WANT TO EXCHANGE BODILY FLUIDS. Furthermore, if you have ANY doubts at all about your partner, you absolutely MUST use a condom and/or a dental dam if you are going to proceed with any of the following exercises. There is no such thing as being too cautious.*

Preparing for Your Orals

An athlete never runs without doing stretches, a boxer never enters the ring without throwing practice punches, and a Bad Girl never gives oral sex without making sure that her oral cavity and the muscles that support it are tension-free. I'm not making this up, folks—this is a true statement! Before you start, you need to loosen up your mouth, jaw, neck, and tongue. Stick your tongue out and make circles with it. Then, open your mouth as wide as you can and stick your tongue out as far as it will go; try to touch your chin with the tip of your tongue. Next, make fish lips; then let your lips come back to a relaxed state. Slowly roll your head around on your neck. Not only will these stretches relax you, but they will allow you to move more freely and be more flexible as you navigate your way around the phallus. This stuff is not a big turn on for guys, so it isn't something he needs to see. But when you're in the bathroom slipping into something "a little more comfortable," do your warm-ups; you'll give the best oral sex of your life!

exercise 10:

The Tongue Lashing

I'm going to assume that you have already given your partner an erotic Zen hand job and that his penis is erect, erect, erect. However, there is no reason why you can't start having oral sex on a penis that isn't erect. In fact, if your guy is a particularly slow *or* particularly fast starter, using the following techniques on his non-erect penis is a great way to get started. The first thing you want to do is use a warm (not hot!), damp washcloth to make his penis (and testicles) squeaky clean. You don't need a mouthful of lubricant, and you also don't need a mouthful of less-than-delicious manhood. Every bit of him should taste great! Your guy will love the attention—it's like having your hands cleaned with one of those little cloths they give you in Japanese restaurants before the food arrives. It adds a special touch.

1. **Begin by licking every square centimeter of the penis.** And when I say lick, I don't mean take sweet little laps like a kitten at a bowl of milk. I'm speaking more along the lines of strong, long licks. The kind of licks you use when you are trying to keep an ice cream cone from dripping on a hot summer day. *Slowly* lick up and down the entire length of the shaft. Make lazy circles on his scrotum with your tongue. Lick up underneath the rim. Flick your tongue back and forth over the opening of the head

of his penis, then widen the circles to include the entire sensitive head. **Use you hands as little as possible at this point.** Not using your hands will force you to chase the penis, giving the activity a very sexy and playful bobbing for apples type feeling. And the way the penis moves this way and that, flopping around, sometimes hitting you in the face if it's erect, is a total turn on—for you as well as him.

2. **Keeping your lips relaxed, slowly take just the top of the head of the penis into your mouth.** You will notice I said mouth. I did not say *vacuum cleaner.* The most common Good Girl misconception when it comes to giving oral sex is that guys like to be sucked on as if they'd stuck their penis down the hose of a vacuum cleaner. This is simply not true. It's called a "blow job" ladies, not a "suck job." Does a woman ever suck the penis when she is giving oral sex? You certainly *can.* But a little suction goes a long way. The concept that oral sex should be *based* on creating suction, and lots of it, is completely misguided. So when you take the head of his penis into your mouth, remember: Take it easy! You can apply some suction, but you're not trying to suck the thing clear off! Just having the head of his penis in your mouth is a lot of stimulation for him, in and of itself.

3. **Flick your tongue back and forth over the top of the head while it's resting in your mouth.** *Ever* so slowly creep your way down the head of the penis with your mouth. Go as slowly as possible, using your saliva to keep him really wet. *Tease him* from time to time by stopping and going backwards for a few seconds. If your man has difficulty becoming aroused, you can suck a little harder. But if he's quick to orgasm, **don't suck at all.**

4. **Continue inching down the length of his penis with your mouth—one slow inch at time.** Use your tongue to play with the penis as you work your way

down the shaft inch by slow inch. You can almost imagine him counting the inches, praying for you to put one more into your mouth. To keep on a delicious edge, slide your mouth up and off the penis entirely from time to time; let it just wave in the air for moment—wanting you. Then slide back down to where you were and prepare to take in another inch. All the time, make sure to keep him really wet with your saliva. For those of you who can't even swallow a single aspirin without gagging, an inch or two of penis in your mouth is quite a lot. Not unmanageable, I hope, but quite a lot—and it may be the place where you have to draw the line. That's okay. A couple of inches of sensitive penis enveloped by your warm, wet mouth is a pretty fabulous thing, as long as you give those few inches a lot of attention. You can simultaneously use your hands to give warmth, comfort, and any necessary stimulation to those parts that are "left out in the cold." Don't make the mistake of avoiding oral sex completely because you don't want to put an entire penis in your mouth—no one sets the rules but *you*.

5. **When you've finally reached the base of the penis with your mouth, begin moving your head up and down the entire length of his penis with slowly increasing speed.** Firmly, but gently grip the penis with your lips and tongue (no teeth!) and keep it really, really wet with your saliva. You might want to grab the base of the penis with your hand (if there's room to get your hand in), or massage his testicles, or both, as you continue to work magic with your mouth.

6. **Alternate stimulating the penis with your mouth and with your hand.** Suck, then stroke, then suck, then stroke. Too much of any one thing, even if that one thing feels pretty great, can still get monotonous enough to decrease his level of arousal. Don't get stuck in a rut doing just one thing the entire

> time; mix up your moves and keep him guessing as to what you'll do next. Unless of course, he begs and pleads otherwise. If you're loving your work, he *will* reach a point where he needs to come. Not *wants* to, *needs* to. Does he deserve his orgasm? Are you going to give it to him? That decision, my Bad Girl, is yours and yours alone.

One other thing worth mentioning before we move on from the topic of oral sex: If giving head is something you normally do with the lights off and the covers pulled over your head, there are a lot of good reasons for you to throw back the covers and keep a soft light on. First of all, you now have oral skills that you can be proud of; show them off! Second, I can't think of *anything* a man likes watching more than the sight of his penis being taken into a woman's mouth. Hmmm. Give me a second here. Thinking, thinking . . . nope, can't think of a damn thing! Finally, when you're "embraced by the light," so to speak, you are actually available for *communication*. You can ask questions like, "Do you like when I lick this?" "How about this?" "Is that too sensitive? Is this too intense?" And, "Who's your mama?" All kidding aside, once you get used to talking to your man while you're handling him, you will find that the awkwardness that can sometimes exist during sex just evaporates. It's totally sexy. Totally grown up. And yes, totally BAD.

Coming Together

You've come, he's come; it's time for you two to come together. I don't mean that *literally*, necessarily, although it has been known to happen! It's time to talk about where you stand, and where *he* stands; and how long he should stand there! In other words, it's time to talk about *sexual positions*, and how they can enhance and intensify your beautiful orgasms.

First, let me say that I have nothing against the standard, face-to-face, man on top missionary position. Although it doesn't allow for the same type of direct and/or intense clitoral and vaginal stimulation that some of the other positions do, the benefits derived from the emotional and psychological connection that can occur when you're face to face with your lover during coitus are, as they say in the commercial, priceless. Can women regularly experience lovely orgasms during sex in the missionary position? Affirmative! I'm among them, I'm happy to say. Sometimes, you just want meat and potatoes, and nothing else will do.

On the other hand, sometimes you want lamb shish-kebab with couscous. Something just a little more exotic. Something like being penetrated from behind, to give just one example. I have no axe to grind with the missionaries, but I can't help wishing that their favored position had been doggie-style instead of the face-to-face entry they made famous! Doggie-style is so much more versatile. First, the woman's clitoris can easily be reached and stimulated with her own hand, with her partner's hand, or with her favorite vibrator (we'll talk about *that* in the next chapter). Second, the man's penis is positioned well to maximize penetration and to stimulate the G-spot and the cervix. And, all that other stuff aside, the purely animalistic quality of the position makes it a very sexy way to screw! But that's just my opinion. You may very well wish that the missionaries had stuck to woman-on-top, or that they'd been creative in a different way!

What are the positions a Bad Girl likes best? That depends on the girl, and on the degree of Bad. Your answer is going to be different from my answer, and it may change as *you* continue to change. But I'm not going to leave you hanging here. In the next few pages I'm going to give you a little starter kit describing the most tried and true. Use your own creativity to build from there.

Getting Well Positioned

CAT: Coital Alignment Technique

CAT is a "kissing cousin" to the missionary position, and requires that the man ride high on the woman while his penis is inside her. This allows the penis and pubic bone to grind against the clitoris of the woman as he thrusts.

- Begin in the standard missionary position. Once inside you, your man should slide up on your body two to three inches, aligning his

178

pubic bone with your clitoris.

- As he begins to thrust, you should feel his penis sliding back and forth against your clitoris. You will also feel pressure on your clitoris and pubic bone from his pubic bone.
- Keep your legs close together. This way you are hugging the penis with your legs, creating even more sensation as your man thrusts in and out. Yow! Don't stop. . . . Don't stop. . . . You are definitely coming!

WOT: Woman on Top

Female is superior! In this position, the woman can control the timing, the depth, the speed, and the thrusting of the intercourse.

- Position yourself so that you are straddling your lover, with one knee on either side of his pelvis. You can either face toward him, or you can face away, toward his feet.
- Insert the head of his penis into your vagina. You can go slowly, as you did in the teasing exercise, or you can sit down on the penis, taking the length of it into you all at once (which can be rather thrilling!)
- Begin raising and lowering yourself up and down on the penis. You can go fast, or you can go slow. Use your finger to stimulate your clitoris while you ride. Then take his hand, and use *his* finger to stimulate you.
- **Squeeze your PC muscle** as hard as you can on the up stroke, or as you slide up on the penis. That will get you where you need to go: the land of the giant O's.
- And don't forget about your breasts. WOT is a great time to give yourself an amazing breast orgasm as you combine all of the sensational erotic elements of this versatile position!

179

REAR ENTRY

A Bad Girl classic. I've already gotten a running start on extolling the advantages of this position. However, to continue:

- Rear entry can be accomplished in a couple of ways. The most common version of rear entry is with the woman on her hands and knees, or on her knees with her butt up in the air. Another variation calls for the man and the woman to lie on their sides, with the man facing the woman's back.
- If your man is standing (as opposed to kneeling) as he enters you from the rear, he will have an amazing range of motion, which can allow him to thrust pretty hard, and vary his strokes more than he usually can.
- *Someone*, either you or he, needs to be playing with your clitoris while all of this is going on. Pulsing your PC muscle in this position brings your G-spot in even closer contact with the penis, which, if you're lucky, can trigger a gusher. Worst case scenario, you just have a real toe curler.

LEGS OVER SHOULDERS

A variation on the male being superior.

- The woman lies on her back. For comfort, or if there is a big height differential between the couple, a pillow or two can be placed under the woman's pelvis.
- The man kneels between the woman's legs. He slides you toward him and tips your hips up a bit in the process. He then places your legs over his shoulders.

- This position is good for stimulating all the hot spots: your G-spot, PC muscle, cervix, and your clitoris. Your breasts and nipples are also free for you to rub, massage, and pinch.
- This position offers all of the psychological and emotional benefits that the standard missionary position does, with the added bonus of allowing for direct contact with the erogenous zones. We're talking about serious orgasm potential here! I give it a ten!

I hope that this chapter has inspired you to be the champion of your own pleasure and of your own orgasms. Let this be just the *beginning* of further experimentation, further exploration, and further investigation into your own body and the sexual pleasure it is capable of providing you. Practice your peaking and plateauing, your Kegel exercises, and your conscious breathing.

It takes twenty-one days to make something a habit; after that, it just becomes automatic. Once practicing those skills becomes automatic for you, you will be well on your way to enjoying a *lifetime* of extraordinary orgasms. I believe you're worth it; don't you?

Chapter 9

Bad Girls Play with Toys

Do you hide your vibrator at the bottom of a drawer, afraid that your lover might find it? Does the thought of buying yourself a dildo make you want to run screaming out of the room? Do you think that couples who use playful restraints as a part of their lovemaking are living on the absolute edge? If you're nodding your head "yes," your Bad Girl makeover is still not complete.

When you were young, you loved to play with toys, but at some time you decided it was time to stop. That's one of the differences between Good Girls and Bad Girls. Bad Girls may have put away their Barbie dolls a long time ago, but they have never stopped playing with toys. Dildos, vibrators, and strap-on harnesses. Ben Wa balls, eggs, love beads, and flavored gels; feathers, furs, blindfolds, and collars. These are just a few of the things you might find in a Bad Girl's private toy chest. Bad Girls have them, love them, and know how to use them. These toys are not just for their own consumption. Maybe when you were a kid, you hated sharing your toys, but every Bad Girl will tell you that the greatest thrill of all comes from sharing their special toys with a man.

Bad Girls love playing with toys in the bedroom. And in the kitchen. And in the den. And in the tub. They know how every toy can add excitement or pleasure, a little extra anticipation, or sometimes a wicked laugh. If you're ready to start playing with toys again too, this is the chapter for you. We'll start with a trip to a neighborhood toy store that's filled with surprises you might not expect. If you have a computer with access to the Internet, we'll also go shopping on-line. I'll teach you the basics, help you get comfortable with your new acquisitions, and give you suggestions for slowly introducing your new toys to your man.

Breaking Free

We've all had times in our lives when we made a decision, or came to a conclusion about something, and we *knew*, right then and there, that our lives would never be the same. It may have been a career decision, or something to do with your personal life—like deciding to move in with your partner or get married. It was big, and you knew your life would change.

You might find what I'm about to say a little funny, but I'm hoping that you have the same kind of watershed experience with this chapter on toys. I hope that in the years to come, you look back on this time and say to yourself, "Wow. My sex life really changed after I read that chapter. What a turning point that turned to be." Because as fun as playing with sex toys is, can, and should be, playing with toys is also a declaration by a woman who takes sex, and her own sexual pleasure, very, very seriously. As you know by now, I want *you* to be a woman who takes sex and her own sexual pleasure very, very seriously.

When you can buy, use, and incorporate some of the sex toys I'm going to be talking about into your sex life (both by yourself and with a partner), you will *definitely* be a very different woman than the one who first opened this book. Sex toys are not for women who are stuck in their little girl. Sex toys are for hot, mature, serious, grown-up women. W-O-M-E-N.

Maybe right now you blush with embarrassment when the word *dildo* is uttered aloud, but after you get finished with this chapter, the only reason you're going to blush is because you're being flooded with sexual heat just from thinking about the pleasure your dildo gives you. Your days of giggling at the words "lubricant," "bondage," or "vibrator" have similarly come to an end. It's ironic that playing with sex "toys" makes you more of a grown-up . . . go figure! But it will; I've seen it happen time and again. Put a small whip in her hand, and all of a sudden Miss Mary Meek becomes Mistress Marian. Don't laugh—it could happen to you!

This chapter is about breaking free from the ties that have been binding *your* hands, and learning how to use those ties to bind somebody else's. No more jokes, jitters, or judgments. It's time for some serious play.

A House Full of Treasures

When you were a kid, you probably had a knack for taking everyday, ordinary, household items and turning them into whatever you needed them to be: An empty oatmeal canister became a castle turret, or a discarded ribbon became a string of pearls. Have you ever heard the expression, "The more things change, the more they stay the same?" Well, here is a perfect example. Because we're going to take that same creative spirit you've always had and bump it up a notch or two.

You will have ample opportunity later on to spend as much money as you want to on all kinds of fancy toys that vibrate, wiggle, tickle, suck, rub, and thrust. But what I'd like you to do right now is just look around your house to see what you *currently* have on hand that might qualify as a bona fide sex toy. There are two excellent reasons to start out this way. First, it will train you to look at the world through sexy eyes, helping you to develop radar for seeing things that could be a source of pleasure for you. Second, why not experiment with what you have on hand, before you spend a lot of money on something that you can already find in your closet, your cupboard, or your crisper?

I don't know about you, but I was a Girl Scout. There are a lot of knots I learned to tie and songs I learned to sing that are distant memories to me, but there's one Girl Scout motto that will haunt me until the day I die: Always be prepared!

The Treasure Hunt Begins

I used to love Sunday mornings when I was a kid. The Sunday paper would come and I would immediately claim the big color comics section for myself. The first strip I would turn to is the one that challenged you to find common, everyday items that were hidden in the elaborate scene being depicted. You might find a lamp, a rope, a flower, a shovel, and a hat, among other things. Sometimes you had to look for a long time, because the artists were really good at camouflaging the objects seamlessly into the background of the scene. Were you a big fan of this kind of comic strip too? Well, it's time to brush up on those object-finding skills, because right now you're going to be picking out everyday items that are being camouflaged by their surroundings once again. This time it's your scene, in your home. And instead of being on the outside looking in, you're going to be part of the scene and part of the action.

Someone's in the Kitchen

Let's begin your search in the kitchen. Go into the kitchen now, then close your eyes for a moment. When you open your eyes again, try looking around your kitchen with Sex-Ray vision. What items do you already have on hand that might lend themselves to a little double duty? Here are some possible kitchen aids for you to consider, and ways to make them even more handy.

Foods

Honey, chocolate sauce, whipped cream, ice cream, ice cubes, mini marshmallows, ripe bananas, strawberry sauce . . . Mmmm. The compliment, "you look good enough to eat," takes on a whole new meaning when you have whipped cream smeared on your breasts! These are just some of the foods that lend themselves to adult sexual play. Have you *ever*? No? Then it's time to find out what you've been missing.

We've all seen movies where food is shown being used in a highly erotic way. *9½ Weeks*, for example (need I say more?). I don't know anyone who doesn't think that the infamous food scene that took place on the kitchen floor in that film wasn't incredibly sexy and exciting. But how many of you have ever tried anything like it? I don't see too many raised hands out there. Well, prepare for a change, because Bad Girls *love* to play with their food. And it's time to assemble your ingredients, get naked, and head for the bathtub.

It's hard to have a food fight by yourself, so if you have a partner who is willing to play with you, by all means invite him to join you. But if you don't have (or want, initially) a partner to join you, it doesn't disqualify you from playing. As you well know by now, a Bad Girl plays with herself all the time!

exercise 1:

Make Your Own Sundae

Since your body may be doubling as a dish for your luscious treats, you want to make sure you're lickably clean before you begin. Taking a hot bath before you start will accomplish this; it will also make the "dish" nice and warm for you for the rest of the exercise. Towel off after you have bathed. Make sure you have all of your ingredients with you.

1. Bring the sauces to room temperature. If you're using chocolate sauce that has been refrigerated, you can warm it first. Pour some into a microwaveable dish and heat on low power, testing the sauce every five or ten seconds until it is *warm, not hot.* Stir it well to make sure there are no hot spots.

2. Drizzle the chocolate sauce over your breasts and chest. Let the warmth envelop you. Ask your playmate to smear the sauce all over your torso, and then lick you clean. Have him touch an ice cube to each of your nipples for a few seconds; get them nice and hard. Next, squirt a couple of dollops of whipped cream just on your hard nipples; let him lick and suck the cream off. You should be feeling

pretty delicious by now! How about a dollop of strawberry sauce in your belly button? Let him get *that* nice and clean, too. A little dab (of something sweet) will do you when it comes to your clitoris. Will it be honey, chocolate sauce, whipped cream? Let him pick his favorite, because you will want him to spend a very long time down there getting every last drop. Best not to get any sauces inside the vagina, of course. (If you do, a gentle douche may be called for later.) If you are playing by yourself, enjoy the way the various textures of the foods feel on your body. Give yourself a breast orgasm with warm chocolate sauce on your chest. Yowser!

3. Time to turn the tables and turn your lover into a fabulous dessert creation. You may want to be a little more careful with the placement of your various foods, since most guys are not too wild about the thought of honey or chocolate sauce in their chest hair. But, by all means, put those dollops of whipped cream on his nipples. During an exercise like this, many men discover that having their nipples sucked and licked is a big turn-on. A lot of women are surprised by how much they like doing the sucking and licking, too.

4. Time now for the penis. Foods don't necessarily make the best lubricants, so I wouldn't try to masturbate him with chocolate sauce or honey. But I would drizzle them on his penis, or paint them on his penis and testicles with a finger or two, and then get busy licking up, down and all around. Be sure to make plenty of "mmm" sounds when you are "eating" him; it will enhance the sensation for both of you. Bon appetit!

Retail Alternative—Flavored body sauces and body paints that come in a boxed set with a brush: $14–30.

Rolling Pin

No, you're not going to hurt anybody, or play out a scene from an Andy Capp comic. A rolling pin can be used to lightly knead out the kinks and knots in your body, and your partner's body, in a fun and surprisingly effective way. A rolling pin can turn you into a brilliant masseuse. It's a great way to unwind before having sex, so that both you and your partner can let go of the stresses of the day and be fully present during sex, giving it all the attention and care it so fully deserves.

---

exercise 2:

Dough Boys

You can use the rolling pin either dry or wet. If you prefer wet, put a little massage oil in the palm of your hand and warm it by lightly rubbing your hands together. With your lover lying on his stomach, apply the oil to his neck, shoulders, arms, torso, buttocks, and legs. Begin using the rolling pin on the shoulders and shoulder blades. Use short back and forth strokes. Be sure to check in with your partner to make sure that the pressure isn't too heavy or too light. Work your way down his body. Change the direction of the strokes as you would if you were rolling out actual dough. I'm in heaven when the rolling pin gets to my buttocks and the *soles of my feet.* Whatever you do, do *not* forget the soles of the feet. Once you've shown him how it is done, it's your turn!

Retail Alternative—Hand-held wooden massagers, sold at bath shops: $14–25.

Feather Duster

Okay, I admit it. I have never intended to use my three feather dusters for housecleaning purposes. My Dust Buster worked just fine. I had an ulterior motive from day one: touching, teasing, and enticing (in that order). The minute I first saw a feather duster at my local hardware store, my Sex-Ray vision showed me what I could do with it. I could just imagine what the feathers would feel like delicately daubing at my bare nipples, my exposed belly button, my naked cheeks . . . and I had a feeling that my lover might enjoy a bit of dusting, too. I was *not* disappointed!

exercise 3:
The Dust-Master

If you or your lover are allergic to feathers, please skip this exercise.

> Start by sprinkling a little talcum or other body powder on the legs, arms, and torso of the recipient (that can be you, or him, or both of you, taking turns of course); powder makes the feathers glide even more smoothly. Begin with the face, dusting oh so slowly. Glide the feathers down and across the collar bones. Dawdle around the nipples. Sweep from side to side, up and down. If you're the recipient of this erotic dusting, part your legs and let the feathers work their magic on the clitoral hood and the vulva. Your partner can watch, or he can dust. (This may be the only time you'll see a guy *beg* to dust.) Dust all the way down to your tippy toes. If you are with a partner, turn over, and let him slowly dust your entire backside.

You can feather dust solo (you might prefer that the first few times), or you can dust with a partner. Either way, it's sure to tickle you.

Retail Equivalent—An erotic feather dusting kit, which includes a small feather duster and edible powder, sold at adult toy stores. $25–30.

Bad Girls Play with Toys

Long-Handled Wooden Spoon

I will bet that you used to consider a spanking to be punishment. I will also bet that you'll feel very differently once you've had your fanny gently paddled during the heat of sex! In fact, you may find yourself shamelessly begging for your partner to paddle you once you've tried it a few times by yourself. A light-weight, long-handled wooden kitchen spoon is a good choice to start with because it minimizes the possibility of too much sting. This is sexy play, *not rough play*. The first time you try paddling, you may also want to protect your bottom by wearing a pair of silky panties. The important thing is to experiment on yourself, first, before you ask a partner to spank you. That way, you can acclimate yourself to the sensation, while maintaining complete control.

---

exercise 4:
Playing the Spoons

There may come a time when a spanking will take you from "zero to sixty" all by itself. I know that for some women, being spanked during foreplay is very effective at getting them aroused. But if you're a novice paddler, start this exercise with a self-caress, and don't start paddling your fanny until you have reached a higher level on your arousal scale (7 or higher). If you associate being paddled with your higher levels of arousal, pretty soon, being paddled will *cause* you to become highly aroused.

> The best position for an erotic self-paddling is face down on the bed (head turned to one side), with bent knees resting on the bed for support, torso raised, and butt up in the air. Start your self-caress. Once you reach a high level of arousal, use one hand to hold the spoon and playfully paddle yourself, and the other hand to seriously masturbate yourself. Rock back and forth and rotate your hips as you paddle and masturbate yourself to orgasm. Bad, bad, bad! And oh, so good!

Retail Alternative—Various whips and paddles sold at adult toy stores: $10 and up.

Back In The Closet

A lot of your clothing and accessories can easily be adapted for use in all kinds of sexual play. Let's take a look now at some of the delightful surprises patiently waiting inside your drawers and closets.

Nylons, Stockings, and Scarves

Someone I'm very fond of gets really turned on when I come to bed wearing an expensive pair of white nylons . . . and nothing else. He loves seeing my pubic hair through the gauzy material and feeling my body through the tight silkiness of the fabric. It feels so naughty!

I know that my friend is not unique in that way. And it doesn't stop at white nylons. As I've mentioned before, earlier in the book, a gorgeous garter belt and real stockings are quite thrilling for most men. Elaborate? No. Expensive? No. Exciting? You better believe it.

But the look is just part of the excitement. Once your partner peels off your sexy stockings, you can use those stockings (or several silk scarves, or a couple of silk ties from *his* closet), to *gently* tie his hands (if you have a two-poster) and feet (if you have a four-poster) to the bed. If you have a "no-poster" bed, you can just tie his hands together. Always use an easy to release bow-style tie; no scary knots and no real hand-cuffs, please! If someone gets hurt or isn't enjoying the game, it not fun. And if it's not fun, it's not play!

This is a good time to slip an *eye mask* over your lover's eyes. One of the many other delightful things you can do while your partner is willingly playing your love-slave is taunting him with the feather duster while his hands are tied. Alternate stroking his penis with the feather duster, and then using your hand. Stroke him again and then use your mouth. Keep switching from your hand, to the duster, to your mouth, to your hand . . . he may never let you untie him! Plus, you'll be putting all sorts of creative ideas into his head when it's *your* turn to be the love-slave.

Retail Alternative—Velcro release cuffs from an adult toy store. $30-$40.

Bad Girls Play with Toys

Costumes and Outfits

I was listening to a local radio station the other day, when one of their more alternative programs came on. I listened to a story being told by a woman who went to a Halloween party this year as a sexy vampire; she and her best friend were wearing collars and being led around on a leash by her friend's husband. It sounded as though this woman had taken a lot of care with her costume, including renting a leather bustier and fastening realistic looking fangs to her eyeteeth. She talked about how the costume changed her personality, and how she enjoyed baring her fangs and hissing at men who looked at her with interest. Some men were *begging* her friend's husband to let them take her leash. Can you imagine? The more she hissed, the more they had to have her. She went on to describe her very interesting and erotic evening.

What special costume or outfit can you imagine wearing that would turn you on in the same way? Is it a naughty nurse? A ranch cowgirl? A cop? Tarzan's Jane? Don't just dream it, do it. Halloween gives us all a great excuse to try on a new persona, but if you have a relationship with someone who's open to the idea of role-playing, why wait till October 31? You can be the trick *and* the treat, tonight! Along with wearing the costume, you can build a whole scene around your character. Maybe your lover would enjoy playing a character, too. He could play a construction worker who comes to the doctor's office for a checkup. The doctor's called away on an emergency and *you* have to conduct the examination. I've got a million of these little scenarios. You do, too. All you have to do is let the genie out of the bottle—actually, that would make a good scenario, too!

Playing a character other than yourself in a sexual situation is really exciting. You may find that you do, say, and ask for (okay, *demand*) things in a way that surprises you. It's like I always say, you've got to dress for sex-cess!

Retail Alternative—Costume purchase or rental from costume shop, toy store, adult toy store, etc.: $30 and up.

A Mirror

Mirror, mirror on the wall, what's the hottest sex of all? Why sex in front of a mirror, of course. We call that dinner *and* a show!

Only the most dedicated hedonists go through the trouble of putting a mirror on the ceiling—and then, only if they don't live in earthquake country! But how about a free-standing full-length mirror? Or one that is mounted on a door –like the one inside of your favorite closet—that can be angled in such a way that you and your lover can watch yourselves at play? A lot of couples get totally turned on and inspired by watching themselves have sex. They often find themselves trying new things just to see how they'll look in the mirror! It's like having your own "blue movie" room.

Are you surprised to see how many ordinary household items—items you may already own—can be easily converted into erotic sex toys? Once you turn on your Sex-ray vision, the whole world will start looking like a giant playground to you. Just remember to always play wisely. Don't put yourself or others in a situation that could end up causing harm. *A Bad Girl may play hard, but she always plays it safe.*

Bring on the Power Tools

A carpenter has her saws, drills, and pliers. A chef has her whisks, pots, and pans. And a Bad Girl has her vibrator, her dildo, and her lubricants. That's just the way it is. A Bad Girl doesn't question the necessity of her tools any more than a carpenter or a chef does—it's impossible to do her best work without them! Sure, when it comes to masturbating, your trusty finger will do in a pinch. But the difference between masturbating using just your finger, and masturbating using some of the fabulous toys that are available to you. . . . Well, it's like comparing a cup of lukewarm, instant coffee from a vending machine that's been lightened with powdered cream, to a piping hot cup of fresh espresso, made with freshly ground beans, which has been topped with a thick, creamy head of steamed milk and a sprinkle of cinnamon—and you're drinking it *in*

Italy! In other words, there *is* no comparison. So fasten your seatbelts— you're in for another wild ride!

In the modern world, there is no shortage of sex toys to choose from for men *or* women. In fact, there are so many varieties of products being offered, your biggest problem is going to be narrowing your choices down to a manageable number of purchases. Let's look at a few of the most popular items that are widely used today, and get you acclimated to the lay of the land.

Dildos

To state it plainly, a dildo is an artificial erect penis. That being true, you would *think* that if you've seen one dildo, you've seen them all. Not exactly! There are probably as many different types of dildos on the market as there are real penises in the world. So if you are a relative newcomer to the wonderful world of artificial erect penises, what in the world should you look for?

Dildo Shapes. Dildos come in myriad different shapes. You can get an anatomically correct dildo with ridges and veins just like the real deal. Some of these artificial penises are ramrod straight, and others are arched in order to have greater contact with your vaginal wall and G-spot. Another popular type of dildo has a head like a real penis, but the length of the shaft is smooth. Some dildos aren't shaped like penises at all. There is, for example, a dildo called the Venus that is in the shape of a *woman's body*. I haven't used this particular dildo, but it is aesthetically beautiful and a best-seller on various websites that offer these wonderful companions.

If you're buying your very first dildo, what shape should it be? You'll know it when you see it. And you *will* see it. In the appendix to this book, I've provided you with a list of stores that offer catalogues and the cyberspace addresses of many fun-to-shop websites that offer a plethora of toys to choose from.

Dildo Sizes. Dildos come in various widths and diameters. Here's one easy way to judge what size dildo might feel best to you: How many fingers do you like inside your vagina when you are aroused? Is it one?

Two? Three? Once you arrive at the answer, *measure* the width of that number of fingers. You will find that most companies that sell dildos through catalogs or on-line quote the diameter of the dildo in their descriptions. Of course, if you can afford to get several different sizes, you can have one for every mood and every stage of arousal.

Length is also an option. If you can only buy one dildo, I vote for a longer one; at least seven inches. You always have the option of inserting only a portion of the dildo, but you can't make it reach seven inches if it's only five inches long. And there are probably going to be times when you will want your dildo to be seven inches long.

Dildo Textures. Most dildos are either made out of silicone or rubber. There are specialty dildos, as I mentioned before, that come in Lucite, or in a new material called *cyberskin*. Rubber is the most bendable substance of all the different types. Sometimes rubber dildos are also referred to as jelly dildos, or dongs. These dildos are softer and more squishy than the other two types. They create a sensation of being filled up, which is very nice, but if they are too soft they may be less effective for vigorous thrusting.

Silicone dildos are the most popular type. They can be a little more expensive than rubber dildos, but they are also more lifelike. Some silicone dildos are hollow sleeves that slip over smooth, cylindrical vibrators, creating five to seven inches of vibrating, almost human, flesh. The most exciting advancement in the world of artificial penises is the invention of cyberskin, which is a material that mimics the qualities of skin so well, you can actually feel the dildo grow warm in your hands. If you were wearing a blindfold, you would swear there was a man attached to it!

Dildo Colors. Dildos come in every color imaginable; some natural, some decidedly unnatural (ever had sex with a bright orange penis before?). *It's your toy, it's your time, it's your choice.* It's *whatever* turns you on. You've taken a pledge not to let the little voices in your head have a say in your decision, remember? Color your world, if you wish.

Bad Girls Play with Toys

Vibrators

Most commonly, a vibrator is used to stimulate the external sex organs, particularly, the clitoris. There are also vibrating dildos and attachments that can be added to some vibrators that make it possible to apply vibration to the entire vaginal canal or directly to the G-spot. As is the case for the dildos, there is no lack of choice in the vibrator department, either. I'm going to stick with the K.I.S.S. (Keep It Simple, Sexy) school of thought and focus on the two most popular vibrator types.

(Magic) Wand Vibrators. A serious appliance. Prices range anywhere from $40.00 to $75.00. A wand vibrator features a large (fist-sized), vibrating head that is attached to a long (eight to twelve inches), slender body that houses the motor. The long handle lends this vibrator a variety of different uses. You can cradle it between your thighs, nestle it between two people, and of course, use it to stimulate your clitoris. Oh, and by the way, it will give you a great neck and shoulder massage as well! Some models accommodate extra attachments such as a G-spot stimulator, a small dildo, or even a vibrating "come" cup for your man.

Coil-Operated or Hand-Held Vibrators. These vibrators are easily obtained, inexpensive, and good at their job. They look like a small hairdryer without the long nozzle. They are smaller and lighter than a wand vibrator, and usually come packaged with a variety of attachments. Compared to the wand vibrator, which delivers a more diffused type of stimulation, the coil-operated vibrator gives a more intense, direct clitoral massage. These types of vibrators typically have two speeds (high and low), though some have a variable speed adjustment. You can find them in the personal appliance section of most major drugstore chains. I'm sure you've seen them before.

Lubricants

I still remember when Dr. Ruth Westheimer brought the word *lubrication* out of the closet and into our homes on her now-famous radio broadcasts. So many people giggled. How could you *not* giggle? But that was then, and this is now, and we all owe the good doctor a debt of gratitude.

I can't say enough positive things about the magic of lubricants. A lubricant can greatly enhance the enjoyment of all sexual activities, especially when using a dildo and other sex toys. When it comes to variety, the sky's the limit. You could literally have your own personal "31 flavors," if you were so inclined. The majority of lubricants designed for use during sexual play are water based, but there are a few that are oil based (these seem to be more popular among fans of anal sex). **A word of caution: If you're using a latex condom, diaphragm, or any other type of latex prophylactic, only use a *water*-based lubricant.** An oil-based lubricant can compromise the integrity of latex.

Some lubricants are thicker, some are thinner. Some are compatible with oral sex, others claim to be edible, but don't taste so swell. One of my favorite websites, *www.goodvibes.com*, has a wide array of lubricants to choose from, as well as good descriptions of their various qualities. If you don't have access to a computer, or if you want something you can use *today*, a visit to your local drugstore or novelty store will provide you with several different brands of sexual lubricants you can choose from.

Playtime Is Now!

I am assuming you now have a vibrator, a dildo, and a lubricant. If you don't have these items, don't pass go, don't collect $200. *Go get your tools!* You're not going to be allowed to graduate with the rest of your class if you don't own the three basic tools found in any Bad Girl's tool chest. Besides, if you don't have the toys, you can't play. And if you can't play, you'll miss out on all the fun!

If you have a computer and you are on-line, the exciting world of sex toys is at your fingertips. If you aren't on-line, you're either going to have to get on the phone or get in your car. I am including an appendix at the back of this book with addresses, phone numbers, and web addresses of some of the larger adult toy stores. Some of these stores will mail you a catalogue if you request it. If you live in a larger city, you may already know of a store that specializes in toys for grown-ups. Don't be shy; take a friend along and go have some fun. All you would really need to buy there is a dildo; everything else you can get at a drugstore, if need be. So go in with a mission, and come out with a dildo (or two or three). But don't be surprised if you come away with a few impulse buys, too; or at least a few new ideas!

exercise 5:

Using Your Vibrator

As always, block out sufficient time to immerse yourself in this exercise without distraction or interruption. *Begin this exercise with a warm bath.* Relax, slow down, and turn your attention away from the outside world and toward your own pleasure, comfort, and peace of mind. Dust yourself with silky powder or apply your favorite body lotion. Be good to yourself; give yourself the royal treatment.

1. Lie comfortably on your bed. Begin with several minutes of conscious breathing. Feel the air relax you even further as it enters and circulates through your body. Use your fingertips in a full-body sensate touch massage. Wake up your body's senses.

2. Turn on your vibrator. Test it against the palm of your hand. Experiment with applied pressure, movement, and speed (if your vibrator has more than one speed). Touch your vibrator all over your body. Put it on your neck, your lips, your nipples. Let yourself get acclimated to the many different sensations it can create on different parts of your body.

3. When you're ready, part your legs and hold the vibrator an inch or two above your clitoris. Slowly lower the vibrator until it just barely touches your

clitoris. Lift the vibrator. Let the vibrations reverberate throughout your body. The biggest mistake most women make when using a vibrator is having a heavy hand. Keep a light touch. Your clitoris is super-sensitive and it's completely unnecessary to go at yourself like a Makita drillmaster. Continue experimenting with this on/off light touch approach. Enjoy the waves of pleasure as they spread through your body like ripples on the surface of a lake.

4. Make circles, stroke the hood of the clitoris, grasp the vibrator between your thighs. Continue touching and stroking with the vibrator until you bring yourself to climax. Some of you may have already climaxed. Congrats! If this is your first time having a vibrator-induced orgasm, I'm sure you see now what all the hoopla has been about! Pretty fantastic, isn't it? And this is just the beginning; there's so much more to "come"!

exercise 6:

Using Your Dildo (with Lubricant)

Carpe Dildum! That's Latin for "seize the dildo." Now that the vibrator has warmed you up and gotten your juices flowing, it's the perfect time to play with your new dildo.

1. First, wash your dildo in warm, soapy water and dry it off. Now, get to know your dildo. Stroke it. Smell it. Lick it all over. Roll it all over your body. Give it a name!

2. Squeeze a generous dollop of the lubricant into your hand. Cover the head and shaft of the phallus with the slippery stuff. Use whatever is left over on your hand to lubricate your vaginal opening.

3. Part your legs and place your feet flat, so that your knees are raised and bent. Clinch and release your

PC muscle several times to relax the vaginal opening. *Very slowly* insert the head of the dildo into your vagina. Allow yourself to feel every fraction of an inch. Once the head has been fully inserted, just allow it to remain there for a few moments. If you had an orgasm using the vibrator, your PC muscle may be spasming lightly around the dildo. Feels good, doesn't it?

4. Pull the head of the dildo out of your vagina. Breathe deeply and let all your muscles relax. If you need more lubricant, go ahead and slather more on. This time, *slowly* slide the dildo a little further into your vagina. Let it rest there as you note your body's response to its presence inside you. Although you may be dying to thrust the dildo in and out of your vagina at this time, resist the temptation for now. Let your arousal grow. After a moment of letting the dildo rest inside you, slide it back out.

5. Continue introducing more and more of the dildo into your vagina. *Take your time.* This is not a race or a competition, it's a process, and the goal is to *feel* as much you possibly can. Feel the ridges inside your vagina as the dildo slides over them. Feel the shapes and ridges of the dildo itself. Once you have worked the entire length of the shaft inside you, just let the phallus rest there against your cervix. Give yourself plenty of time to fully enjoy the terrific sensations. You're in control of this experience; make the most of it!

6. Just as slowly as you worked the dildo *in*, you are going to do the same thing in reverse, as you work the dildo *out* of your vagina. *Slowly* inch the dildo out and back, out and back. Each time, slide a little more of the dildo out, before you slide it back in. Think of your cervix as being home base and allow the head of the dildo to rest there every time you slide it back in. Which feels better—inching the

dildo in, or inching the dildo out? Or are they equally fabulous? How often do you get to go this slowly when there is a man controlling the penis? Not too often, I'll bet.

7. Once you have inched your dildo all the way out of your vagina, you have had a proper introduction to your newest toy, and I encourage you to experiment with various thrusting speeds and motions. Unlock your hips and move them around while you are thrusting. Be sure to use plenty of lubricant; if your thrusting motions become intense, the lubricant will protect you from chafing or drag due to friction. Keep breathing. Relax your body. Have a bunch of fabulous orgasms.

"I'll Have the Combo Platter, Please . . . "

Once you are comfortable with the basics, here are a couple of toy combinations you can try:

Combination #1: Dildo, Lubricant, and PC Squeezes.

When you are withdrawing the dildo after a deep thrust, **squeeze your PC muscle as you slowly pull the dildo out.** In other words, *contract* the PC muscle on the down stroke (the exit stroke). Try to keep your surrounding muscles relaxed. Each contraction not only strengthens your PC muscle, but brings you closer to an exquisite orgasm.

Combination #2: Dildo, Lubricant, and Vibrator

This variation is the equivalent to a sex toy triple play. Lubricate your dildo. Slide your feet toward yourself so that your legs are bent at the knees. Part your legs. Slide the well-lubricated dildo into your vagina and begin a gentle thrusting motion. Hold your vibrator with your free hand. Begin to apply light, short, strokes and touches to your clitoris with the vibrator as you continue thrusting with the dildo. Use your plateauing technique to see how long you can last before you give in to **one of the best orgasms of your life!**

Other variations to try include squeezing your dildo between your legs while you use your hands to bring yourself to a breast orgasm. Or use the feather duster in tandem with your vibrator. You can go as far as your imagination (and your energy level) can take you.

Make a Play-Date

I often hear friends of mine who have children talk about the play-dates they arrange for their kids. Sometimes I wonder about the formality of the practice when it comes to kids, but I think it's a marvelous idea for any *adults*. Adults are likely to go weeks, months, and maybe even years without ever having a date with another adult that is specifically set aside for the purpose of sexual play.

It's time for you to have a play-date. Half the fun of having a new toy is being able to share it with a friend, don't you agree? When you arrange for your date, you can let your playmate know that you've bought some new toys for the bedroom that you could use his help assembling. Guys love a technical challenge!

Some women worry about the reaction they might get from a man if they introduce a vibrator or a dildo during sex. Before you worry too much, let me tell what usually happens: You barely have time to pull the thing out before it is in the very willing hands of a very excited partner. In fact, does the term "opening the floodgates" mean anything to you? Most men figure that sexual toys are strictly taboo—that is, unless the woman introduces them first. Then it's as if someone has just called for recess in the middle of a history exam; I'm talking playtime pandemonium. So go forward with confidence.

exercise 7:

Play Time

Have all your tools within easy reach of the bed. These tools include, but are not limited to at least one dildo, a vibrator, and a couple of different types of lubricant. You should also have several latex condoms.

Variation #1

The first time you use a vibrator in bed with your lover, start with "show and tell." Lie on your back and give him a live demonstration of the way you use the vibrator on yourself. Show him how much pressure he can comfortably use and how long he can keep the vibrator on your clitoris. Let him experiment with it while you give him lots of verbal feedback (including your "oohs" and "ahhs," of course).

Once he has the hang of it, smear some lubricant on his finger and glide it into your vagina. If you have a small dildo, he can use that instead. Have him continue to use the vibrator on you as he *gently* and *slowly* thrusts his finger or the small dildo in and out of your vagina. If handling both the vibrator and the dildo is too much of a challenge for him at this point in time, then *you* hold the dildo, or use your own finger while he continues to excite you with the vibrator.

Some women enjoy having a finger or dildo inserted into their anus, too. If you are among them, just make sure you have *lots* of lube on the item that is to be inserted. **Never put an object that has been in the anus back into your vagina (or any other orifice) without first washing it thoroughly.** This includes the human finger. Don't take chances with your health!

If you have been lying on your back, try turning over and assuming the modified rear-entry position, with your head and shoulders on the bed, and your butt in the air. Your lover can reach between your legs with the vibrator, or he can reach around from the side. This position also allows you to continue thrusting with the dildo. If you feel the clitoral stimulation is becoming too intense, don't be afraid to ask him to stop for a while, or alternate to very short "taps" with the appliance. Of course, we would all love for you to have an earth-shaking orgasm, but sometimes our bodies need some time to adjust to a new type of stimulation. What you don't want to do is over-stimulate the clitoris, or suffer from clitoral burn-out. Remember, tomorrow is another day!

Variation #2

Here is another way to use a vibrator with a partner.

Assume the rear entry, or doggie-style position. Slather your lover's penis with lubricant and let him slowly slide it into your vagina. While he is thrusting inside you, masturbate yourself with the vibrator. Use a light, short touch. Then, reach a little further back and *lightly* (please!) touch the vibrator to his *testicles*. He probably won't be able to withstand more than a few seconds of this kind of stimulation at a time; it's sure to feel pretty intense to him. Check in with him—ask him how it feels. Continue to alternate applying the vibrator to him, and then to you.

You can also use this technique while you are sitting on top of your partner. As he thrusts up into you, or as you slide up and down on his penis, reach behind you from time to time to touch his thighs, testicles, and entire pubic area with the vibrator. Then reach back around and use the vibrator on yourself. Squeeze your PC muscle periodically, especially as you feel orgasm approaching.

Continue switching back and forth from you to him to you with the vibrator. Squeeze the PC muscle *hard* when the orgasm hits; it's sure to send you both into paroxysms of pleasure.

Variation #3

Here is a vibrator technique to use on him that will have him eating out of the palm of your hand, and anywhere else you want him to be eating . . .

Begin by slowly licking your lover's penis. Grab the penis at the base, and alternate licking, sucking, and hand stimulation. When his penis is half to fully hard, wrap one of your hands around as much of the penis as you can. Pick up and turn on the vibrator with your other hand. *Press the vibrator head* (if it's a wand style), *or the vibrator body* (if it's a coil operated style), *against the back of the hand that is holding his penis.* The vibrations will travel through your hand and up his gorgeous member.

Now, continuing to hold the vibrator against your hand, *take his penis into your mouth.* Hold his penis in your mouth and feel the vibrations going through your hand, through his penis, and into your tongue and lips. So sexy! Slowly bob your head up and down on his vibrating shaft. Take his penis out of your mouth and lick the length of it from time to time. Give light squeezes with the hand that is holding him as the speed of your stimulation increases. When he's breathing heavily, moaning, and close to orgasm, *take the vibrator away every five seconds for a five-second interval.* When you re-apply it, it will feel even more intense to him and it will very quickly push him over the top into a climax. Oh, you naughty girl!

And this, as they say, is just the tip of the iceberg. The more you engage in relaxed play with these and other toys, the more variations you will discover, invent(!), and enjoy.

The Exotics

Now that we've covered the basics, let's take a look at some of the more exotic toys that you may decide to add to your collection.

Vibrating Eggs and Butterflies

A vibrating egg is an egg-sized, egg-shaped vibrator that comes in either metal or plastic. Many models allow you to control the speed at which the egg vibrates via remote control; the egg is attached by a long cord to a small box that holds the batteries. An egg can be held in your hand and placed wherever you want it on the body. The egg can also be placed in a harness that is worn around the waist, which holds the egg against your clitoris. This allows you to enjoy constant stimulation of your clitoris while you're making love, or when you are simply in the mood to feel good all day.

Bad Girls Play with Toys

Butterflies are similar to eggs in that they are small vibrating devices that nestle up against your clitoris. However, they differ from eggs in that they do not lend themselves to be being used anywhere except in the vaginal area. Some of them come pre-attached to a belt, and others must be held in place. Butterflies are smaller eggs, and if your desire is to wear a vibrator during the day (can you imagine!), you may find them easier and more discreet to wear underneath your clothes.

Ben Wa Balls and Other Objets du Sex

Ben Wa balls have a long and illustrious history. Opinions are divided between Ben Wa enthusiasts and others who say that it is much ado about not a lot. A Ben Wa ball is actually a ball bearing—it is about the size of a large marble, and it contains a smaller metal ball within the outer ball. When the Ben Wa balls are inserted into the vagina (slowly and carefully), and you walk around or masturbate, they create a subtle vibration that (many women claim) amplifies the sensations of pleasure.

There are also other types of balls that can be inserted into the vagina. Some of these variations are connected by latex-coated string, which makes it easier to pull the balls out when you are ready. The sensation of the balls being slowly pulled can be extremely pleasurable in and of itself.

Whips, Slappers, and Swatters

If you or your partner find that getting paddled with a wooden spoon just leaves you wanting more, you can upgrade to all sorts of exotic apparatuses that take spanking to a whole new level. Keep in mind, though, that when you are standing over someone with a whip in your hand, or vice versa, it is obvious that an element of domination has been introduced to your sexual play. The first time you engage in this kind of play with your partner, it's probably a good idea to lay down some ground rules *before you begin*. Ground rules such as: how hard is too hard, how long is too long, and "If I say stop, we stop." You must be in *complete* agreement about this. The last thing either of you wants to do is to go too far and scare, or hurt, the other. However, once you are both clear on your boundaries and you are feeling comfortable, safe, and secure, you may find that a combination of light "whipping," role-playing, and costuming provides you and your lover with hours of sexual excitement.

Anal Plugs, Probes, and Beads

If you are a Bad Girl who enjoys anal penetration, you have a veritable excess of choices. From thin, thick, to thickest, to ridged, waved, curved, and spiraled, there is a butt plug and anal probe for every personal preference and whim. Some even come with a suction cup so that you can stick them to the floor or the wall and inch your way down on it to your hearts content. All anal products need to be used with a lot of lubricant. This is especially true for anal beads, whose devotees state that the balls give more pleasure upon departure than on arrival.

Anal stimulation isn't just for women, either. Many men enjoy stimulation ranging from a finger circling the rim of the anus, to actual penetration. It's equally exciting for many women to *give* pleasure in this way. If it's something that you would like to explore, stop *wondering* if it's something he would like: *ask* him.

Erotic Videos

Videos can be a source of inspiration, education, and stimulation. There is a myth that says that women don't get sexually aroused through visual stimulation. Like hell! In my many years as a sex therapist, I have found that the great *majority* of women I work with become highly aroused while watching a sexually explicit movie or reading sexually material. They may have a hard time *admitting* it at first, but once they understand that it is common, normal, and natural, most of them have a great time integrating the use of videos into their sex lives.

Some adult videos are like mainstream movies, with involved plots, character development, and high-quality production values. Other videos are more "cinema verité," with an almost homemade quality to them. Other "educational" videos (actually, I find all videos educational) show you how to have better sex with your partner, how to perform certain sex acts, or how to have a "gusher." Today, there are as many videos that are filmed for a woman's enjoyment as there are for a man's enjoyment. Many times, the two are interchangeable—depending on what you enjoy. An increasing number of videos are created intentionally for couples, carefully attending to the erotic needs of men *and* women.

Bad Girls Play with Toys

There is as much variety in the world of adult videos as there is in all of the other categories of sexual entertainment. And you don't even have to traipse down to your local video store anymore. Many of the websites that are included in the appendix of this book sell or rent videos on-line. They also offer reviews, ratings, and descriptions for each one. So if you've never indulged in the pleasure of watching sex on film, there is simply no reason not to. It isn't one-size-fits-all anymore; there are adult films out there just for you.

If you don't already have a fabulous toy chest to hold all of your fabulous toys, run, don't walk, to your nearest Pier One, Cost Plus, or even your local thrift store, to find a chest (preferably one that locks) to keep your goodies in. Buy a *big* one, because toy chests are like closet space: The more space you have, the more you will buy to fill it up! So what are you waiting for? School's out, you Bad Girl! Go home and play!

Chapter 10

Bad Girls Break All the Rules

Your transformation is almost complete. The Good Girl who opened this book at page one is now a tiny figure in the rear view mirror of your car, getting smaller and smaller each moment as you leave that predictable, uninspired sexual past behind and head full throttle into the exciting, powerful, sexually connected world of Bad Girl sex.

What will your sexual future look like? For the first time in your life, you probably don't have a clear answer to that question. And that, my friend, is a very good thing. It tells me you are on the threshold of an exciting new beginning.

You see, for years and years you knew *precisely* what your sexual future was going to look like: It was going to look exactly the same as your sexual past. Sex, for you, had become completely predictable. Gratifying at times, with special moments here and there perhaps, but far from thrilling and far from memorable. If you ever had sexually thrilling days and sexually memorable days, they were now firmly cemented in the past tense. And if there was any direction your sexual world was traveling, it was the direction of decreasing expectations and evaporating enthusiasm.

Maybe you had hopes and dreams that some sexual miracle would occur—that your body and its full sexual potential would magically open up to you one day through some life-changing event on a moonlit beach thousands of miles from home. Or that a knight in shining armor would come galloping into your world one day (in his 300 horsepower high-performance driving machine), sweep you off your feet, and carry you into a world where you would feel ignited and excited. I know all about these hopes and dreams. I also know that, if you are like most women, you had probably stopped giving a lot of energy to these fantasies any more. More likely, you had entered into the acceptance phase of your sexual development; the phase where you have accepted the fact that the giddy, heady days of sexual thrills are gone for good. Time to find excitement in other ways. Time to move on. Time to take up gardening.

But now all of that has changed, hasn't it? Some simple exercises, some new information, and already, you have discovered a reservoir of sexual energy waiting for you inside of yourself, and a big "Welcome Home!" sign lighting up your sky. You didn't need a man to make this happen, and you didn't need a miracle to make this happen. All you had to do was give yourself permission to reclaim what you have always held deep inside of yourself; permission to reclaim the Bad Girl within.

So now you feel BAD. Truly BAD. You look BAD, you think BAD, you walk and talk BAD. You touch BAD, you tease BAD, you play BAD, and you have the BADDEST, most beautiful orgasms you've ever had in your life. And you feel so darn good about it it's hard to believe that it's really you. But it *is* you. All you. And all so wonderfully BAD.

When You're Trying Hard to Be Good, Sex Is One Long Waiting Game

When it comes to sex, Good Girls always play by the rules—a long list of rules about what is and what is not appropriate sexual behavior. Rules about when you can have sex, how you're supposed to have sex, and how much sex you're supposed to have. Rules about who gets to be on top and who gets to have the first orgasm. Rules about what you can ask for and how many times you can ask. Rules about what you can say and how you can say it. Rules about what you can touch and how much you can touch it. Rules about what is taboo and what is tasteful. The rule book is thicker than the Manhattan phone book, and it is equally mind-boggling.

Overwhelmed and overburdened by all of these sexual rules and regulations, Good Girls find themselves frozen solid—afraid to make a move, afraid to rock the boat, afraid to be too sexual. That means Good Girls do a lot of waiting. A lot of waiting for HIM . . .

- Waiting for HIM to want you.
- Waiting for HIM to get turned on.
- Waiting for HIM to take the lead.
- Waiting for HIM to touch you.
- Waiting for HIM to excite you.
- Waiting for HIM to ignite you.
- Waiting for HIM to make you feel good.
- Waiting for HIM to break new ground.

Waiting, waiting, waiting. I can get pretty miffed just thinking about it. We have all wasted so much time waiting—waiting for something that we had in our possession all along.

What do you see *now* when you look at this list? Does it make you want to laugh out loud? Can you see now how crazy it has been to live your life this way? Can you see how much *work* you were doing to be a Good Girl? That kind of work is absolutely exhausting. No wonder you had so little enthusiasm for sex! No wonder you had so little energy!

Now, the Wait Is Over

That was then, this is now. You had your reasons for being so good. But now you have a book full of reasons for leaving that passionless world behind. Your moment has arrived. It's time to break all those old rules.

Being a Bad Girl puts an end to the waiting. Once you have stepped inside that powerful sexual center you have no reason to wait any more. You are in control now. You know what you want. You know what feels good. You know how to get there. And you don't need *him* to do anything but sit back and enjoy the show.

The Good Girl's Guide to Bad Girl Sex

I haven't spent a whole lot of time in this book giving you detailed explanations of sexual acts. I haven't offered thousands of sexual positions to keep your lovemaking fresh, I haven't given you a plumbing manual to enhance your understanding of male anatomy, and I haven't led you through Tantric sexual secrets that can extend an orgasm for hours or days. I haven't done this for a reason. Tons of books have already been written about this kind of stuff. Heck, I have written half a dozen books about this kind of stuff. The information is out there, and you can find it in any bookstore. What you *won't* find, however, is a guide to charting your own sexual course, a guide to breaking rules and breaking taboos as it suits you in the service of having the most dynamic sex. Why? Because the only person who can guide you there is *you*.

In the first nine chapters of this book I have given you the secrets to discovering your own power. And now, in this final chapter, it is my pleasure to give you the last, most precious secret that the Bad Girls know—the secret to using that power for the rest of your sexual future. That secret is only six words long: **you have to break the rules.**

A Lifetime of Sexual Surprises

One of the most important signatures of Bad Girl sex is that it is totally unpredictable. It never looks the same way twice. It never feels the same way twice. It never starts the same way twice. It never ends the same way twice. That's the most delicious part. Because part of being Bad is being able to constantly surprise your partner, and, far more important, being able to constantly surprise *yourself*.

Bad Girls are constantly surprising themselves. They are surprising themselves with the intensity of their sexual appetites, with the intensity of their sexual curiosity, with their openness to experimentation, with the intensity of their arousal, with the intensity of their orgasms. They are surprising themselves with their own sense of abandon, with their limitless sexual energy, with their sexual passion. And they are surprising themselves with their ability to ignite passion in their lovers. That is what happens when you leave the world of the Good Girls behind and root yourself firmly in Bad Girl turf.

Stepping into Your Sexual Future

One door closes, another door opens. And the door that has opened for you is the door to your sexual future—a future without limits.

How often will you have sex? Maybe three times tonight, and then not again for the next two weeks. Maybe three times tonight and three times tomorrow. Maybe twice a night for the next two years! How often will you masturbate? As often as you need to, to keep your internal sexual connections fully charged. Every morning, or every night, or twice on Saturdays, or all of the above! Will you experiment with different positions? If that turns you on. And maybe they won't look like anything you've ever seen in an illustrated manual. Maybe you'll be lying on the dining room table, completely naked, feeding yourself turkey and mashed potatoes with your fingers while your lover is filling his mouth with you. Or maybe you'll be taking a luxurious bubble bath with your lover kneeling beside the tub so he can keep his penis in your mouth. Or maybe you'll be lying on your stomach comfortably in bed, watching the evening news—only you're naked from the waist down and your lover is delivering his special evening headlines with furious abandon. When you are breaking all the rules, every day is different and every sexual moment is different.

Does that sound BAD, or what?

Going, Going, Gone!

So I ask you one last time: Are you ready to break all the rules? Are you ready to say goodbye to the restrictive, controlling, spirit-crushing, libido-crushing stuff that has ruled you life for way too long? Are you ready to live your life on a more erotic edge? Are you ready to never, ever be Good again? I think you are. I think you are feeling so excited by what you have already discovered inside of yourself that you are ready to leave your sexual past behind and *never* look back. I think you are more than ready.

So congratulations, graduate! You are no longer a Bad-Girl-in-training. Starting today, you are the genuine article. Toss your graduation cap high in the air, pop open the bubbly, and give yourself a toast. Today *is* the first day of the very best part of your life. You are finally one-hundred-percent W-O-M-A-N, and thoroughly, unmistakably BAD.

215

Appendix

Shop Till
You Drop

GOOD VIBRATIONS
(http://www.goodvibes.com)

By far, this is my favorite website for all things sexual on the Internet. For one thing, it's a great-looking site; there is absolutely nothing tacky or distasteful about it. Good Vibrations is also owned, run by, and fashioned for women. It features a spectacular array of products and informative descriptions of them all. They also let you know which products are the favorites of their customers and their staff. Good Vibrations has two retail stores, and they're happy to talk to you if you call with questions:

> 1210 Valencia Street (at 23rd Street)
> San Francisco, CA 94110
> 415-974-8980

> 2504 San Pablo Avenue (at Dwight)
> Berkeley, CA 94702
> 510-841-8987

For a catalogue, call them at: 800-289-8423.

TOYS IN BABELAND
(http://www.babeland.com)

A very cool, very fun site. If you live in New York City or Seattle, Washington, you're in luck, because they have retail outlets there. The rest of us can visit them on the Internet or call them for a catalogue for at-home shopping.

> *94 Rivington Street*
> *New York, NY 10002*
> *212-375-1701*

> *707 E. Pike Street*
> *Seattle, WA 98122*
> *206-328-2914*

A WOMAN'S TOUCH
(http://www.a-womans-touch.com)

Home of the female-shaped Lucite dildo I referred to in the toys chapter. This site may have the most amazing array of dildos on the Internet. Oh, and if you're a midwestern Bad Girl, get ready for a day trip, because this is within driving distance!

> *600 Williamson Street*
> *Madison, WI 53703-450*
> *608-250-1928 or 888-621-8880*

ADAMEVE.com
(http://www.adameve.com)

As the name implies, this site is geared toward both sexes. AdamEve.com also offers a *lot* of different types of cyberskin dildos. You can even take a virtual *pinch*! Don't ask me how they do it, you've just got to see it to believe it.

To order by phone or request a catalogue: 1-800-293-4654

3 WISHES LINGERIE
(http://www.3wisheslingerie.com)

Interested in role-playing but don't know where to begin? Begin here! This site has an extraordinary array of costumes to wear when you're in the mood to act out. You can buy the costumes from them, or just spark your own ideas!

> *7909-125 Falls Of Neuse Road*
> *PMB 172*
> *Raleigh, NC 27615-3348*
> *919-844-8515*

Sorry—they don't offer a catalogue at this time.

LINGERIE-SHOPPING.com
(http://www.lingerie-shopping.com)

For your more everyday, run of the mill . . . hot, hot, hot, killer lingerie items. This site has something for every woman, lots of sizes, and nice large pictures of everything they sell.

They offer several catalogues: 1-800-990-5519

FEMME EROTIC
(http://www.femmerotic.com)

The subtitle for this site is, "The Pro Sexual/Pan Sexual Independent site network." In other words, this is an eclectic mix of fascinating articles, erotic stories, and links to other sites on the Web. Have fun!

Index

221

Index

KY Jelly, 119

Labia, 116
Laughter, 143
Learned helplessness, 20
Legs Over Shoulders, 180
Librarian, 27
Licking, 174
Lingerie, 47. *See also* underwear
LINGERIE-SHOPPING.com, 219
Listening skills, 94
Look, 44. *See also* presentation
Lubricants, 119, 170, 198, 202, 204

Makeovers, 64
Makeup, 6, 56, 63
Massages, 148, 189
Masters and Johnson, 120
Masturbation, 101, 150, 162, 169, 205
Mealtimes, 36
Memories, 18-19
Messages, 14
Midday Direct-Dial, 146
Mirrors, 194
Misconceptions, 11
Mission statement, 17
Missionary position, 178
Mixed messages, 44, 49, 90
Mons veneris, 116
Morning Handful, 144
Mouth, 133
Myths, 11

Nipples, 162, 181
Nylons, 192

Obscenity, 12
Oral sex, 108, 173
Orgasm, 39, 41, 110, 123, 150, 153

Paddles, 207
Panties. *See also* underwear
PC muscles, 38, 179, 180, 181, 202
Peaking, 156
Peek-a-Boo, 145
Penises, 167
Perineum, 118
Pheromones, 81
Physical appetites, 10

Plateauing, 156, 203
Play dates, 203
Pornography, 12
Positions, 124, 178
Power, 23
Prepuce, 117
Presentation, 30, 68. *See also* look
"Prick tease," 141, 148
Promises, 142
Pubic
    bone, 116, 122, 179
    mound, 168
    triangle, 116
Pubococcygeal muscle. *See* PC muscle
Pussy, 124

Rape, 16
Rear Entry, 180, 205
Recklessness, 12
Relationships, 13
Reprogramming, 11
Restraints, 183
Rolling pins, 189
Rules, 213

Satisfaction, 9
Scarves, 192
Scrotum, 168, 174
Seduction, 127, 140
Self
    consciousness, 108
    control, 11
    expression, 102
    esteem, 11
    paddling, 191
    touch, 73, 129, 136
Sexual
    abuse, 16
    appetites, 9
    boundaries, 27
    categories, 26
    development, 9
    hunger, 10
    positions, 177
    power, 2, 8, 14
    techniques, 9
    thoughts, 25
Shame, 6, 8
Shaving, 47

223